P9-DIG-202

DATE DUE

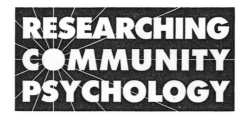

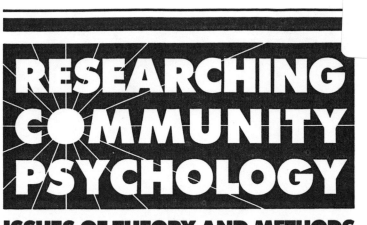

ISSUES OF THEORY AND METHODS

EDITED BY

**PATRICK TOLAN,
CHRISTOPHER KEYS,
FERN CHERTOK**
AND
LEONARD JASON

**American Psychological Association
Washington, DC**

Published by
American Psychological Association
1200 Seventeenth Street, NW
Washington, DC 20036

Copies may be ordered from
APA Order Department
P.O. Box 2710
Hyattsville, MD 20784

Designed by Paul M. Levy
Typeset by BG Composition, Baltimore, MD
Printed by Arcata Graphics Book Group, Landover, MD
Technical editing and production coordinated by
Theodore J. Baroody

Library of Congress Cataloging-in-Publication Data
Researching community psychology: issues of theory and methods/edited by Patrick Tolan . . . [et al.].
   p.cm.
   Papers from a conference sponsored by the APA Science Directorate and held Sept. 9–10, 1988, at DePaul University. Includes bibliographical references (p. 229) and index.
   ISBN 1-55798-098-5
   1. Community psychology—Congresses. I. Tolan, Patrick H. II. American Psychological Association. Science Directorate. RA790.55.R47 1990
   362.2'042'072—dc20 90-972
Printed in the United States of America.
First edition

CONTENTS

CONTRIBUTORS

LaRue Allen, *University of Maryland, College Park*
Meg A. Bond, *University of Lowell, Massachusetts*
Brenna H. Bry, *The State University of New Jersey—Rutgers*
Cary Cherniss, *The State University of New Jersey—Rutgers*
Fern Chertok, *Newton, Massachusetts*
William S. Davidson II, *Michigan State University*
Maurice Elias, *The State University of New Jersey—New Brunswick*
Stephen B. Fawcett, *University of Kansas*
Carolyn L. Feis, *U.S. General Accounting Office, Washington, DC*
David Glenwick, *Fordham University*
Kenneth Heller, *Indiana University*
Barton J. Hirsch, *Northwestern University*
Stevan E. Hobfoll, *Kent State University*
Leonard Jason, *DePaul University*
James G. Kelly, *University of Illinois at Chicago*
Christopher Keys, *University of Illinois at Chicago*
Cynthia Kingry-Westergaard, *University of Illinois at Chicago*
Murray Levine, *State University of New York at Buffalo*
Jean Ann Linney, *University of South Carolina*
Raymond P. Lorion, *University of Maryland, College Park*
Kenneth I. Maton, *University of Maryland, Baltimore County*
Edward P. Mulvey, *Western Psychiatric Institute and Clinic, Pittsburgh,
    Pennsylvania*
J. Robert Newbrough, *Vanderbilt University*
Kenneth I. Pargament, *Bowling Green State University*
Bruce D. Rapkin, *New York University*
Julian Rappaport, *University of Illinois at Urbana–Champaign*
Thomas M. Reischl, *Michigan State University*
N. Dickon Reppucci, *University of Virginia*
Stephanie Riger, *Lake Forest College*
LaVome Robinson, *DePaul University*
Edward Seidman, *New York University*

Irma Serrano-García, *University of Puerto Rico, Rio Piedras*
William R. Shadish, Jr., *Memphis State University*
Marybeth Shinn, *New York University*
Carolyn F. Swift, *Wellesley College*
Ralph W. Swindle, *Stanford University School of Medicine*
Patrick Tolan, *DePaul University*
Edison J. Trickett, *University of Maryland, College Park*
Abraham Wandersman, *University of South Carolina*
Roger P. Weissberg, *Yale University*
Allan W. Wicker, *The Claremont Graduate School*

FOREWORD

Federal research agencies stopped regularly supporting investigator-initiated "state-of-the-art" research conferences in scientific psychology well over a decade ago. Yet, over that same period, scientific psychology has continued to grow—as well as to diversify into many new areas. Thus, there have been relatively few opportunities for investigators in new and cutting-edge research areas to convene in special settings to discuss their findings.

The American Psychological Association (APA), as part of its continuing efforts to enhance the dissemination of scientific knowledge in psychology, undertook a number of new initiatives designed to foster scientific research and communication. In particular, the APA Science Directorate, in 1988, initiated the Scientific Conferences Program.

The APA Scientific Conferences Program provides university-based psychological researchers with seed monies essential to organizing specialty conferences on critical issues in basic research, applied research, and methodological issues in psychology. Deciding which conferences to support involves a competitive process. An annual call for proposals is issued by the APA Science Directorate to solicit conference ideas. Proposals from all areas of psychological research are welcome. They are then reviewed by qualified psychologists, who forward substantive suggestions and funding recommendations to the Science Directorate. At each stage, the criteria used to determine which conferences to support include relevance, timeliness, and comprehensiveness of the topics, and qualifications of the presenters. In 1988, seven conferences were funded under this APA Science Directorate program's sponsorship, and seven conferences were funded in 1989. We expect to fund six more in 1990, at an annual overall program expense of $90,000 to $100,000.

The APA Scientific Conferences Program has two major goals. The first is to provide, by means of the conferences, a broad view of specific topics (and, when appropriate, to provide for interdisciplinary participation). The second goal is to assure timely dissemination of the findings presented by publishing a series of carefully crafted scholarly volumes based, in part, on each conference. Thus, the information reaches the audiences at each conference as well as the broader psychological and scientific communities. This enables psychology and related fields to benefit from the most current research on a given topic.

This volume presents findings reported at the September 1988 conference, "Researching Community Psychology: Integrating Theories and Methodologies." It attempts to outline some of the crucial issues facing community research—epistemological issues, the nature of the relationship between the researcher and the "researched," how to balance conceptualization and statistical analysis, and so forth. In the manner of a conversation, moreover, it attempts to articulate some "criteria of excellence" and to consider the very meaning, processes, and results of a continually evolving area of research. In addition to community psychology researchers, scientists of other perspectives lent their voices to the discussion, including developmental, organizational, and behavioral psychological researchers.

This volume is representative of what we at the American Psychological Association believe will be a number of exceptional volumes that give readers a broad sampling of the diverse and outstanding research now being done in scientific psychology. We hope you will enjoy and be stimulated by this book and the many others to come.

A list of the conferences funded through this program follows:

Researching Community Psychology: Integrating Theories and Methodologies, September 1988
Psychological Well-Being in Nonhuman Captive Primates, September 1988
Psychological Research on Organ Donation, October 1988
Arizona Conference on Sleep and Cognition, January 1989
Socially Shared Cognition, February 1989
The Role of Experience in Modifying Taste and Its Effects on Feeding, April 1989
Perception of Structure, May 1989
Suggestibility of Children's Recollections, June 1989
Best Methods for the Analysis of Change, October 1989
Conceptualization and Measurement of Organism–Environment Interaction, November 1989
Cognitive Bases of Musical Communication, April 1990
Conference on Hostility, Coping/Support, and Health, November 1990
Psychological Testing of Hispanics, February 1991
Study of Cognition: Conceptual and Methodological Issues, February 1991

Lewis P. Lipsitt, PhD
Executive Director
Science Directorate, APA

Virginia E. Holt
Manager, Scientific Conferences Program
Science Directorate, APA

PREFACE

This book constitutes a conversation about the developing scientific enterprise of community psychology research. It is an attempt to articulate and to punctuate critical issues and to consider conscientiously the intent, process, and products of community inquiry—to integrate the "tender" interests in bettering social welfare and in humanizing the communities and settings in which we live with the "tough" value of methodological discipline that can build a reliable, utilitarian body of knowledge.

This is not a "how to" handbook, although specific research methods (e.g., Chapters 11 and 13A–E) and recommended practices (e.g., Chapters 14 and 15A–E) are presented. It is not a compendium of exemplars, although several illustrations of "good" community research are mentioned (e.g., Chapters 2 through 7 and Chapter 16A–D). It is not a philosophical treatise, although philosophical implications are frequently emphasized (e.g., Chapters 3, 8, and 16A–D) and specific stances are advocated by several of the authors (e.g., Chapters 4, 6, and 16A–D). Instead, this book represents a discussion among active researchers about the nature of their shared endeavor of community inquiry and about the issues that concern them as they follow this interest. Thus, the authors address issues from the most abstract, such as the nature of scientific knowledge, to the most pragmatic, such as how to disseminate results. In this conversation about community research, the contributions do not speak in unison nor are they intended to build, each on the previous one, to collectively instruct the reader. Pieces addressing the same issue often present different perspectives or opposing views. Few controversies are settled. Many are articulated for the first time, some are "thickly described" to promote a shared meaning of what the problem with which we are wrestling is, and some are developed toward finer distinctions and more complex evaluations. The coherence of the conversation is not in what is said about what to do; rather, it emerges in an agreement of the need for careful consideration of research aims and processes. In sum, the purpose of this book is to stimulate thought about the process of community research as a scientific enterprise. We hope that this stimulation can guide the reader toward producing more satisfying, useful, enriching, and adventuresome research.[1]

The book is one outcome of a conference sponsored by the American Psychological Association (APA) Science Directorate and held September 9 and 10, 1988, at DePaul University in Chicago. The conference was jointly supported by funds from the Science Directorate and by financial and in-kind contributions from the hosting psychology departments of DePaul University, the University of Illinois at Chicago, and Roosevelt University. Over 80 invited researchers, students, and leading contributors to the field from academic institutions and agencies from across the United States attended.

For two days, the conference focused on four major topics for conducting community research: key concepts and theoretical approaches, hypothesis generation, issues in analysis (especially concerns in studying the person *and* the setting), and implementation. The conference was organized so that each topic was addressed through a three-step sequence, consisting of a presentation to the whole group, followed by small-group discussions convened in order to reflect and to build upon the whole-group presentation, and concluded by a reconvening of the whole group to synthesize information generated in the small groups. The framework for the small groups, as well as the goal of the synthesizing meetings, was to offer *criteria of excellence,* or recommendations that each presenter or group would offer about how our research work should be done. These recommendations sometimes took the form of suggested standards, sometimes were presented as challenges to the field, and sometimes took the form of important questions to be addressed. The hope was that this format would nudge the field toward expression and clarification of the qualities of research conception, design, and implementation that we, as a scientific community, consider desirable. This book is intended to increase the likelihood of that nudge occurring. The conference and the book represent an outgrowth of both the maturing of the field as a contributor to scientific psychology and the concurrent frustration with the constraints of the predominant model for psychological research.

Although the contents are disparate at times, the book's coherence emerges in the flow of the conversation across topics. The conference and the book were organized to focus on the major topics that we encounter, even if we do not recognize them, each time we undertake research. These topics are addressed in the order in which they are usually addressed in actually conducting research. As in any good conversation, addressing each topic may mean raising more questions or may involve refining or complicating the questions used to start the conversation. Each topic, then, can be organized by the questions raised about it.

---

[1]The term *adventuresome research* was contributed by Jim Kelly in a preconference planning meeting. It captured the spirit of the often-expressed dilemma of community researchers, in which they feel that their interests in action conflict with the methods commonly accepted in psychology. Constructing new or additional methods and a different perspective that support careful but adventuresome approaches to the dilemma became a central theme of the conference and is mentioned throughout this book.

ORGANIZATION OF THE BOOK

As indicated above, the book focuses on four main topics. The title of each of the four corresponding major parts refers, first, to a general experimental science descriptor and, then, to a specific community psychology issue. Each topic discussion is organized around a set of prompting questions, whose central goal is to develop criteria of excellence. Because the first question for most scientists is to ask how to determine the worth of one research question versus another according to a given theory, the book begins (after an introductory essay by the editors) with William Shadish's discussion of an approach to evaluating the importance and robustness of a research endeavor and the questions driving that research. He provides a framework for evaluating the theory and the methods that guide our work. He also begins what is a common occurrence in the subsequent chapters: generating questions that community psychologists need to ask themselves and that the field needs to discuss regularly.

Part Two, Key Concepts: Approaches to Framing the Endeavor, addresses questions about how theories can contribute to our research and about the role of theory in community psychology research. Each of the first five chapters addresses these questions by speaking about a theory or concept that has been highly influential in community research. Some describe how existing theoretical approaches can enrich community psychology—developmental (Lorion), organizational (Riger), and behavioral (Fawcett)—whereas others explain the implications of values and theories primarily developed within community psychology (Rappaport and Kingry-Westergard and Kelly). In each part, stimulus chapters are followed by a criteria-of-excellence chapter or chapters that discuss issues raised in the stimulus chapters. In the first discussion chapter (Chapter 8), Glenwick, Heller, Linney, and Pargament identify common assumptions and tensions that cross the five preceding chapters. In addition, they lay out several possible future directions for theory building within community psychology.

Part Three moves the focus to hypothesis generation, with questions concerning the purposes of hypotheses, how they should be generated, and how much we should strive to bring together multiple perspectives in generating these hypotheses. Seidman presents a conceptualization of social regularities as the phenomenon of interest that can bridge the diverse interests of community psychologists by providing a method of generating hypotheses. This is followed by a discussion chapter by Bry, Hirsch, Newbrough, Reischl, and Swindle on the epistemological issues in hypothesis generation, the ability of the field to realize its goals in hypothesis generation, the general implications of attempting to focus on social regularities in generating hypotheses, and other criteria-of-excellence concerns.

The chapters in Part Four are organized around an extended examination of the central and thorny methodological issue of levels of analysis. As presented by Shinn in Chapter 11, this issue provides a conceptual, measurement, and analysis-technique problem that affects most community psychology work. This chapter is followed by one consisting of five conceptual analyses of the implications of Shinn's examination and of the topic of interest in multiple levels of analysis in general. These responding conceptual analyses are organized by the question of how this approach evaluates multiple-level phenomena and the issue of context. Each conceptual analysis—behavioral (Elias), ecological (Wicker), empowerment (Davidson), organizational (Cherniss), and developmental (Allen)—takes a specific viewpoint that corresponds to the five conceptual views used to present the theoretical frames in Part Two. Chapter 13 is a collection of brief evaluations of methodological approaches and issues. Each section of this chapter is organized around the implications of multiple levels of analysis for a particular methodology topic. Thus, Rapkin and Mulvey (quantitative), Maton (qualitative), and Levine (historical analysis) each focus on one analytic method, with an emphasis on evaluating multiple-level phenomena. Reppucci and Hobfoll each address similar implications for two important validity criteria (ecological and conceptual).

Part Five focuses on the issues of implementing our research, which for community psychologists is a matter of actualizing our values in our research design and in our method of working with the community on research. This part is organized by the questions of how our research designs can take into account the values of collaboration and action and how our dissemination efforts should reflect our values. Serrano-García presents a blueprint for conducting community research in a manner that is congruent with the values of community involvement and assuming community competence. She challenges us to consider the process of our work as much as the product. Five examinations of subtopics or related issues to the process of doing our research then provide, in a criteria-of-excellence chapter, a compendium of brief analyses of topics (Bond on entry, Weissberg on fidelity and adaptation, Wandersman on dissemination, Robinson on data feedback and communication to the host setting, and Swift on intervention effects of research).

The final major section (Part Six) provides a series of evaluations and perspectives on the topics discussed within the book and on the conduct and impact of community research. Chapter 16 provides the perspectives of four active participants in such work (Feis, Cauce, Trickett, and Shadish), each of whom is at a different point in his or her career. The final chapter integrates the numerous views and criteria suggested within the book. In keeping with the spirit of the rest of the book, this integration is intended less as a reliable guide than as a stimulus to spur the reader toward thoughtful research that generates questions and ideas that will allow enrichment of the field and provide useful encounters with community psychology interests.

Similarly, the areas of research that are discussed, the perspectives that are presented, and the questions that are raised throughout the book are provided as means of organizing and of spurring on the conversation that is community psychology research. Our intent is to enable, not to constrain. We hope that this volume will aid you in contributing to the conversation.

Patrick Tolan   *Christopher Keys*
Fern Chertok   *Leonard Jason*

ACKNOWLEDGMENTS

Preparing this book has been an exciting and rewarding exercise in collaboration with the sponsoring universities, the American Psychological Association, and the community of authors. This feeling of an exercise in community psychology was true not only in the sense that this is a collection of contributions, but also in the investment that the conference participants and authors brought to the planning and preparation of the conference and to their chapters. We have been lucky to have worked in a responsive, caring, and industrious community. We believe this occurred because, just as we were motivated by our felt need to converse about the topics involved in carrying out community research, there was a consensual base of interest and recognition of the topics' timeliness across much of the field. In other words, the interest was not particular to us, but arose concurrently for many others, so that participants brought heightened interest to the task. Thus, even more than in most edited volumes, we must acknowledge the extent to which this book is the result of considerable effort by a large group of colleagues.

In addition, we want to specifically thank Doreen Koretz for encouraging this undertaking, Jim Kelly for his help in conceptualizing the conference agenda, Ray Lorion for his continued sensible counsel, and Steve Johnson for his tireless editorial assistance. The Departments of Psychology at DePaul University, the University of Illinois at Chicago, and Roosevelt University, Dr. Marjorie Piechowski and the Office of Sponsored Programs and Research at DePaul, and Virginia Holt and Alan Kraut of the American Psychological Association Science Directorate enabled this work to be produced. The secretarial staff of DePaul, especially Lucinda Rapp, provided excellent support and remained patient throughout the ever-expanding requests made of them. All have our gratitude and should share in the credit for any beneficial impact that this work may have.

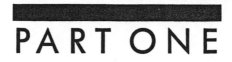

PART ONE

OVERVIEW

CHAPTER 1

CONVERSING ABOUT THEORIES, METHODS, AND COMMUNITY RESEARCH

PATRICK TOLAN, FERN CHERTOK, CHRISTOPHER KEYS, AND
LEONARD JASON

Psychology . . . affords a spectacle of science still in the making. Scientific curiosity, which has penetrated so many of the ways of nature, is here discovered in the very act of feeling its way through a region it has only begun to explore, battering at barriers, groping through confusions, and working sometimes fumblingly, sometimes craftily, sometimes excitedly, sometimes wearily, at a problem that is still largely unsolved. (Heidbreder, 1933, p. 425).

Since its inception over 20 years ago (Bennet, Anderson, Cooper, Hassol, Klein, & Rosenblum, 1966), community psychology has developed into a flourishing field that is a major contributor to psychological science, an essential part of many graduate training programs, and a vibrant research interest shared by a community of scientists. Emerging from clinical, social, developmental, organizational, and experimental psychology, the research endeavors of community psychology have been grounded in applying sound methodology to wrestle with "real world" problems and to develop alternative solutions for those problems. As often noted, it is a field that struggles constructively with the tension between rigorous methodology and the values of social action (Cowen, 1980; Keys & Frank, 1987; Lorion, 1983; Munoz, Snowden, & Kelly, 1979).

    Conferences on community psychology have served to catalyze development of the field through important steps toward the concerns prompting the Chicago conference that is the basis of this book. The Swampscott conference in

1965 examined the limitations of then current training and research models and defined the initial direction of the field and the roles of community psychologists. The 1975 Austin conference examined training issues and emerging models for training. The 1980 Tampa conference focused on the issues of training in terms of community psychology as an independent academic endeavor. In 1987 the occurrence of the First Biennial Conference on Research and Training in Community Psychology signified the maturing of a vigorous research field. The success of the recent 1988 conference, from which this volume was generated, demonstrated that community-oriented psychological research is a common interest that both cuts across subdisciplines within psychology and influences adjacent disciplines. These developmental markers of the field indicate a level of maturity that calls for an evaluation of community psychology as a research endeavor. The ensuing evaluative discussion articulates and reviews the field's scientific status by examining current theories, methods, and implementation issues.

The 1988 Chicago conference was also prompted by constraints that were felt in applying traditional scientific research design principles to community research. As is exemplified by its oxymoronic title, community psychology is interested in the person in context and the context in persons. Conceptually, this interest requires moving beyond a goal of context-free theories of behavior, trait-oriented measurement, and reductionistic research designs taken from traditional laboratory psychology. In its germinal stage, community psychology retained many of the trappings of a traditional positivistic scientific model, causing several evaluators to note that the field's work was not on a par with its rhetoric (Loo, Fong, & Iwamasa, 1988; Lounsbury, Cook, Leader, & Meares, 1985; Novaco & Monahan, 1980). Subsequently, as community research proliferated, a number of questions arose about the applicability of the philosophy, principles, and practices of traditional research to the problems and questions of interest to community psychology (e.g. Kingry-Westergaard and Kelly, this volume; Seidman, 1983). It is still the case that, although some consideration is given to community and multidisciplinary methods in graduate training, traditional methods are usually emphasized more strongly and distinguished as primary in the enterprise of "science." Little consideration has been given to the underlying assumptions driving such methods and to the implications that such assumptions have for the knowledge that can accrue. To date, the lack of a forum for a formal exchange about these concerns has left community psychology researchers to construct individual unsatisfactory solutions. Some researchers have been prone to rely blindly on traditional research, whereas others have rejected scientific inquiry in general, without critical evaluation of the explanatory viability of traditional principles.

Recognition that this set of choices was unacceptable coincided with the maturation of the field in such a way as to attest to the need for a focused discussion among colleagues about the field's research status. This need to converse also reflected a view of the form, process, and goals of our research: knowledge construction as a conversation. As this book progresses, many topics, strategies, dilemmas, and needs will be discussed. Less articulated than the explicit viewpoints advocated in each chapter, but running throughout the book, is the premise that, because knowledge is contextual and constructed, the information of value to community psychology is more in the nature of enriching ideas, in new and more complex questions, and in the shared meanings of the field than in the uncovering of elemental phenomena. Thus, the metaphor of a conversation provides a useful framework for the field, and certainly for this book's organization and purpose.

SCIENCE AS A CONVERSATION: A PERSPECTIVE ON ITS FUNCTION AND ITS RELATION TO COMMUNITY PSYCHOLOGY

This book argues for setting our scientific endeavors apart from the purpose and process of science as it is borrowed from 18th-century Newtonian physical sciences (Fiske & Shweder, 1986; Popper, 1968). This borrowed model has a "root metaphor" (Pepper, 1970) of mechanistic causality. One corollary of this metaphor is a reductionistic explanatory process that attributes greater "truth" to elementary phenomena than to more complex or molar phenomena. The model also assumes that these elementary phenomena are universal and that they are true across all phenomena studied. The goal of a science of this nature, then, is to isolate a single requisite cause (Chaplin & Krawiec, 1979; Mitroff, 1983; Popper, 1968).

These characteristics conflict with community psychology's emphasis on the contextual nature of information (Kelly, 1984; Riegel, 1976), the utility of divergent views and solutions (Rappaport, 1981; Seidman, 1983), and the need to emphasize how our work is done as well as what is done (Chavis, Stucky, & Wandersman, 1983). These values raise questions that are not easily addressed by a traditional model of scientific knowledge. For example, what epistemology is adequate for the complexities and dynamism of community phenomena? What new ideas and conceptual frameworks are needed to identify, elucidate, and understand these phenomena? How do these new ideas help investigators frame research questions? How can a science of individuals take the setting and the individual–setting interactions into account? How can researchers develop effective collaborative relations with other researchers and with community members, and how should these relations be understood as part of what is studied? What is the relationship between action and knowledge? How is the social context of knowledge to be considered?

Given the traditional model's limited applicability, it follows, then, that the "normal science" activity (Kuhn, 1970) of incremental building of knowledge by a group of researchers, all working on a few big questions within a single, shared theoretical orientation, is an inauthentic description of community psychology, both now and in the future. The main thrust of most of our work has been and continues to be toward articulating divergent perspectives on community

phenomena and developing shared connotations and denotations of the terms that
we use to represent the phenomena of interest (e.g. Heller, Price, Reinharz,
Riger, & Wandersman, 1984; Sarason, 1981). Such a thrust not only indicates
the basic interest in developing a shared symbol system (McMillan & Chavis,
1986), but also indicates the personal investment of the researchers and their
shared utopian vision (Kirkpatrick, 1986; Rappaport, 1977). This view translates
to attempting to evaluate theories (see Chapters 3–8, this volume), construct
taxonomies (Frederickson, 1972; Moos, 1984), analyze methodological issues
(see chapters 9, 11–13, this volume; Susskind & Klein, 1985), and clarify our
conception of community (Hunter & Riger, 1986; Kirkpatrick, 1986; McMillan
& Chavis, 1986).

This conflict in purpose with the traditional model of scientific knowledge
is not considered simply a reflection of the early age and "preparadigmatic"
status of community psychology (Kuhn, 1970), but rather reflects an essential
nature of our field of inquiry as a social science (Cronbach, 1982; D'Andrade,
1986; Shweder, 1986). For these reasons, and assuredly for many others, it is
unlikely that community psychology, as could be said of most social sciences,
will shift radically toward one shared view as the result of a groundbreaking
experiment or some accumulation of pieces of knowledge. As noted by Cronbach
(1986), "social science is cumulative, not in possessing ever-refined answers
about fixed questions, but in possessing an ever-richer repertoire of questions"
(p. 91).

Several explanations of what distinguishes community psychology's interests from those of a traditional scientific research model can be put forth. For
example, community psychology tends to be interested in "ill-structured" problems, whereas the traditional scientific model is designed for work on well-
structured problems (Churchman, 1971; Mitroff, 1983). Ill-structured problems
are distinguished from well-structured problems in that the latter tend to be
solvable if the right sequence of steps is used in applying set principles. The
problem is viewed as the same from all perspectives, and once solved, the
solution is applicable to the problem whenever it is encountered. Ill-structured
problems tend to be those that do not have well-defined or reliable methods of
determining what the problem is and how to solve it. As is true of most problems
of interest to community psychologists, the problem definition varies depending
on which stakeholder's perspective is used (Seidman, 1983). The relation of
knowledge to action is not reliable across encounters with the problem. Ill-
structured problems require regular but differing solutions depending on where
and when they are encountered. Thus, the goal of deriving context-free universal
causes and, therefore, final determined solutions is irrelevant. A more useful
goal is to attempt to develop more enlightening and enriching questions about
and descriptions of the problem.

Another explanation of what distinguishes community psychology's interest
may be that, by emphasizing the variation in problem definition according to
setting, perspective, and time, we are indicating inherent valuing of the subjec-

tive, while divorcing that valuing from rejection of scientific analysis and logical (objective) evaluation. This view has been termed *divergent rationalities* (Shweder, 1986). Shweder argues that what may appear from the outside, on the basis of values driving an outsider's logic, to be an irrational belief or matter of faith, from the insider's view may have a logic or rationale that is consistent and quite defensible. He suggests that this is the situation underlying the thorny philosophical problem of the essential contestability of any social science explanation. A divergent rationalities view suggests not only valuing and applying different responses to problems, but also striving to produce a diversity of questions and answers. As has been noted by others, community psychology's interests are in matters that are best understood by multidimensional analysis of systems, rather than by identifying a single causal element (Cook & Shadish, 1986; D'Andrade, 1986; Gleick, 1987). If diversity is endemic to the study of the phenomena that we are interested in, there can be no knowing apart from the stakeholder's position and the theoretical and historical context. Yet, from that position, a defensible, scientifically logical (partial) description can be provided.

Thus, our knowledge is not a matter of uncovering, but rather one of conversing in an increasingly complex and enriching discussion. The research products constitute an ever-larger compendium of information and insights about community phenomena. These views suggest a root metaphor of a *conversation* to organize our "normal science" activity.

From this view, then, the purpose of community psychology research is to construct knowledge as shared understanding that permits "useful encounters" with the phenomenon of interest, rather than that of discovering of postulated forces and entities existing independent of the investigator's conceptual viewpoint (Cronbach, 1986; Seidman, 1983). Thus, the field's scientific character can be defined as the development of descriptors that are treated as "real" for the sake of conversation. The process of the scientific work is exchanging descriptions and enriching the meaning of actions (whether that is achieved by intended intervention or intended evaluation). This is a contextual and constructivist philosophical stance that emphasizes that "nonlogical necessities"—primary values, stakeholder position, utopian vision (Kirkpatrick, 1986; Shweder, 1983)—determine the rules for "rational" inferences and the "logic" we rely on in our day-to-day scientific business (Mitroff, 1983). The value of research knowledge, then, is in its descriptive richness, explanatory utility, and conceptual robustness, rather than in its situational independence, ability to prove a general fact, and generalizability of results. This view of research as the conversing of like-interested (but not necessarily like-minded) scientists looks for coherence and explanation in patterns rather than consistency of results and conclusions (Gleick, 1987; Seidman, this volume).

In applying the conversation metaphor to the work of community psychology research in this book, we hope to articulate further the general role of theory in research, as well as the implications of specific theories. We hope to deritualize methodologies so as to reconnect them with the theories and concepts instigating the inquiry. Taking such a view means rejecting a choice between an objective versus a subjective orientation by giving subjectivity a hard look and noting the soft side to "objective" information (Shweder, 1986). It also means acknowledging and evaluating the political and social processes of carrying out community research. It means taking an action with the awareness that it is only one of several viable actions that could be taken (Rappaport, 1981). From this view, the values of the researcher are overtly expressed by the research design as well as by the rhetoric used to interpret findings. It means more conscious use of methods and theories with the goal of enlightening rather than establishing cause and effect (Cook & Shadish, 1986). This book strives to provide a conversation that advances our awareness of the questions that we are asking and highlights promising methods for enriching our repertoire of questions.

CHAPTER 2

DEFINING EXCELLENCE CRITERIA IN COMMUNITY RESEARCH

WILLIAM R. SHADISH, JR.

This book addresses the issue of criteria for excellence in community research. That issue is just one step short of the larger question of what is good science. No one has provided a satisfactory answer to that question in over two millennia. Hence, we ought to approach this task with a good deal of humility about the prospects for succeeding. Yet there is a certain logic that we can follow in addressing the topic. This logic stems from what philosophers refer to in ordinary language as *analysis of valuing* (Rescher, 1969; Scriven, 1980). They claim that whenever we make value statements about anything—this is a good car, a good book, or good research—we engage in certain steps that we can call the *logic of evaluation:*

1. Select criteria of merit—those things that would have to be done if a thing were to be called *good;*
2. Set standards of performance about how well the thing being evaluated would have to do on each criterion;
3. Measure performance on each criterion; and
4. Synthesize the results into a summary statement about the merit of the thing being evaluated.

A familiar example is evaluating an automobile in the manner of *Consumer Reports* testers. They ask what the car would have to do to be good and how well it would have to do it, they measure each car's performance on each criterion, and then they combine the results into a statement about which car is best. It

9

does not matter if we are making value statements about automobiles, food, or community research—the formal logic is the same.

This book is most obviously about the first step in this logic: selecting criteria of merit in community research. So the bulk of this chapter will be about that step. However, at the end of this chapter, I will briefly consider the other three steps.

THE STARTING POINT: WHAT SHOULD COMMUNITY RESEARCH DO?

The logic of evaluation says that we need criteria of merit. We can get them by asking what it is that community research does, and what it should do. There is no single right answer to this question. Many of the differences that might divide community psychologists in their understanding of good work may stem from basic differences in their understanding of the nature of the field. Therefore, each of us must explicitly state our vision for the field, so that we can consider these differences.

One might start by asking if there is anything special about community research that would require different criteria of merit than those that might be appropriate for related fields such as program evaluation or policy research. On the whole, I hope that there are no differences that are important enough to overcome the common ground among these specialties. Despite their differences, these specialties all share the goal of producing useful knowledge about the worth of different ways of addressing social problems. This vision of community research is broad in the interdisciplinary sense, and accords no special respect to the particular history of community psychology. The criteria I will discuss are aimed at facilitating this broad vision: addressing social problems.

However, it would be naive to think that there is nothing at all special about community psychology. It has its own developmental history, in which certain values and concepts have gained currency, and it has a special concern with the notion of community that gives many researchers a sense of unique identity. Any discussion of criteria for excellent community research that does not recognize these special features risks falling on deaf ears. But such risks may be worth taking for researchers who are committed to addressing social problems in the broadest sense. For such researchers, the special features of community psychology are not always compatible with this broad concern because they often involve accepting restrictions in the kinds of interventions studied and not studied, in the levels at which one intervenes, and in the methods and concepts that one uses in doing so. To be sure, this vision of social problem solving is sometimes compatible with traditional visions of community research—but sometimes it is not, and then the researcher has to choose between the two visions and try to justify the choice.

I take heart that my particular vision is not entirely idiosyncratic, because it seems that some community researchers are themselves ambivalent about the extent to which "community" ought to be the dominant metaphor for the field. For example, the very first *Annual Review of Psychology* chapter on the topic—and all chapters since then—was not titled "Community Psychology," but was more broadly titled "Social and Community Interventions" (Cowen, 1973). Although this broader label undoubtedly has many sources, I suspect it partly reflects the wisdom of those who do not want to limit their challenge too much. Furthermore, sound epistemological reasons exist for not ossifying the special features of a field of study. As we become more secure in the newfound maturity of community research, we can afford to look outward to different ways of doing and thinking about the research. Indeed, we must do so if we are to grow.

It should be a matter of debate, of course, which vision of the field is best. But such visions must be made explicit as a prerequisite to understanding the differences among us in the criteria of excellence that we then propose. My criteria stem from my understanding of what I want community research to do.

CRITERIA OF MERIT FOR COMMUNITY RESEARCH AIMED AT SOCIAL PROBLEM SOLVING

The phrase *criteria of excellence* elicits a notion of specific prescriptions about things that community researchers should and should not be doing. A good example is Campbell and Stanley's (1963) famous dictum that internal validity is the sine qua non of good research, implying that we should all strive first and foremost for internal validity. The problem with this approach is that we have yet to find many (if any) such prescriptions that hold always and everywhere. Hence I prefer to think in terms of more flexible criteria (criteria of merit) that might best be characterized as realistic, well-reasoned, informed, and tailored answers to the key problems that impede our efforts at addressing social problems. The answers are realistic to the extent that they recognize the real-world constraints about which the experience of the past 20 years has taught us. They are well-reasoned to the extent that they do not violate plausible standards of thinking and evidence without good explanation of why the violation is warranted. They are informed to the extent that they take into account the major alternative constructions on the topic. And they are tailored in the sense that they are situationally bound to particular problems or circumstances rather than being generalized prescriptions.

In my experience, there are four key problems that impede our efforts at addressing social problems and that, therefore, require realistic, well-reasoned, informed, and tailored answers:

1. How does social change occur?
2. How is scientific knowledge used in social change?
3. What do we do about values and valuing?
4. What is going to count as knowledge?

There will often be no single correct answer to these four questions. Rather, each question often points to a problem in which each of the available options has some advantages and some disadvantages. Given this condition, it is important to ensure that the answers provided by each particular theory are chosen with a high degree of consciousness about available alternatives and that none of the disadvantages are shared by all available paradigms without our being aware of this constant bias and choosing to allow it to remain unaltered.

There is a fifth problem that I will not discuss, given space constraints: How should we do research in a way that takes into account our answers to the first four questions, yet is still practical given the constraints under which we work? The answers to this fifth question are what I call *theories of research practice* (Cook & Shadish, 1986). Theories of practice tend more toward practical, specific advice about such things as which questions to ask, which methods to use, and what roles the researcher should strive to fill. These are the questions to which most researchers need immediate answers as they go about the day-to-day implementation of research. Theories of practice are essential to scientific work and are more immediately useful than discussions of abstract matters such as ontology, epistemology, or the nature of values. Many of the approaches and paradigms that are considered in this volume are probably best thought of as theories of practice. Still, each theory of practice, either implicitly or explicitly, must assume an answer to each of these four questions, so that the worth of the theories of practice depends on the worth of those assumptions. By discussing the first four problems, therefore, I hope to suggest a framework against which we can think about the worth of the theories of community research practice that follow in this volume. My discussion of these four problems is necessarily brief and distilled from my past work (Cook & Shadish, 1986; Shadish, 1984, 1986b, 1987).

Social Problem Solving and Social Change

The first set of problems facing community researchers concerns the nature of social problem solving and social change. The problem is that social change of a meaningful kind is very difficult to achieve. One reason is that the more important the social problem, the more difficult it is to solve, because, by definition, important problems tend to involve more people, more money, and more vested interests. A second reason is that the bigger the proposed intervention, the more likely it is to have big effects, but the less likely it is to be feasible. A third reason is that, although interventions are more implementable if they are consistent with the beliefs and structures of the system that has to implement them, the more consistent an intervention is with the system, the less likely it is to be different enough to make a real difference.

In the context of such difficulties, the problem is that, if you want the change to actually happen in the short term, you mostly have to think small—you must deal in small problems, small interventions, small adjustments to what is already being done, and small effects. At some point, however, thinking small defeats the purpose of social problem solving—some things change, but the problem-generating ideologies and structures functionally stay the same. Thinking big in all these matters avoids this problem, but is extremely unrealistic if the goal is short-term change, because the structures and ideologies are not present to support any radical change. It is the rare intervention that succeeds at being both implementable in the short term and functionally important. The frontiers of good theory on this topic are here, helping us to recognize interventions that are both widely implementable and important at the same time (Shadish, 1987). For example, the phenothiazine medications were probably important contributions to ameliorating the problem of major psychotic disorders, but were also implementable because they fit well into the medical model underlying service funding and distribution.

When I judge the merits of a piece of community research, therefore, I look to see, first, if it explicitly recognizes this trade-off between implementability and importance, and, second, whether it implicitly seems to favor implementability or importance in the kinds of problems and interventions that it studies. If it displays no awareness of these issues, then it is likely to contribute to social problem solving mostly by accident. Unfortunately, I rarely see good discussions of these matters in community psychology. But there are exceptions. The text written by Heller and his colleagues has an excellent discussion of social change; and Seidman's *Handbook of Social Intervention* has the virtue of multidisciplinary treatment of social problem-solving issues. Good journal articles on the topic include Weick's (1984) article on small wins and Sarason's (1978) article on the nature of social problems. However, we could profit greatly by looking outside community psychology to work by political economists, for example, Lindblom's *Politics and Markets* (1977, 1983; Manley 1983; Shadish, 1987).

Use of Research in Social Change

The second set of problems faced by community researchers concerns research utilization. Traditional disciplinary training tells us little about how to do research that is more likely to be useful in social problem solving. The omission is glaring if we believe that applied social research should be both useful and used. The merits of a theory of research should, therefore, be judged by consideration of the following matters in regard to its assumptions about the usefulness of the research that it recommends doing: First, is the theory clear about to whom it wants to be useful, and does it provide a reasonable and explicit justification for its prioritization of users? Different users tend to want different things, and it is rarely possible to serve them all. Second, is the theory clear about the kind of use that is sought? In answering this question, it is helpful to differentiate between instrumental use, conceptual use, and persuasive use (Leviton & Hughes, 1981). Instrumental use is the use of research results to dictate direct changes in programs; conceptual use aims to change the way that people think about problems and their solutions; and persuasive use tries to marshall convincing evidence to support a particular position. Third, what does the theory recommend about what the researcher has to do to facilitate use? In particular, are those recommendations appropriately tailored to the kind of use desired? Different kinds of use require

very different tactics. For example, instrumental use is best facilitated by identifying key decisionmakers and using them in planning the research, limiting the
study to variables that can be changed, communicating research results early and
quickly, and writing short reports with action recommendations. Conceptual use,
on the other hand, resembles basic social research in that none of the preceding
tasks is addressed; but there is a more conscious effort than in basic research to
change the way that people think on the issue by seeing that the findings travel
through the relevant networks of program staff, blue-ribbon commissions and
panels, mass media, interest groups, and academic issue networks (Weiss, 1988).

The trade-offs about use closely resemble those about social change. That
is, facilitating instrumental use of research, especially in the short term, tends to
require focusing studies on decisions and improvements that will usually make
only a minor difference in important problems and that, at worst, result in trivial
findings subordinated to the interests of the most powerful groups. Focusing on
conceptual use allows us to address problems and solutions that can more successfully and radically change the way people think about issues, but it also
usually results in research of no immediate instrumental use to anyone.

If a theory of community research does not consider these matters, or says
things that clearly violate what the past 20 years of field research have taught us
about how research gets used, then one cannot be hopeful that the resulting
research will be useful. In the past 10 years, community psychologists have
begun to struggle with these issues. For example, efforts to develop collaborations with the persons or groups being studied are often partly justified on the
basis of making research useful to those with a stake in the program being studied
(stakeholders). But some "reinventing of the wheel" could be prevented by
greater familiarity with the voluminous literature on research utilization. Sociologist Carol Weiss has written extensively on the use of social science by policymakers (Weiss & Bucuvalas, 1980) and presents some of the best discussions of
doing research to facilitate conceptual use (Weiss, 1978, 1988). Conversely,
Michael Patton has written extensively about methods for facilitating instrumental
use (Patton, 1986, 1988b). There is also the possibility of misuse of research
(Cook, Levinson-Rose, & Pollard, 1980) and that a latent effect of research can
be to stifle change (Stake, 1986). Finally, Lindblom and Cohen's (1979) treatise
on *Usable Knowledge* is a superb statement about the role of information relative
to other political and economic interests in decision making.

Community Psychology and Values

The third set of problems concerns the role of values and valuing. When judging
the merits of a community research theory, it is important to study its justification
for its choice of which values to represent in the study. Notice that this problem
is not merely that a good theory should simply have values. All community
research implicates values. Rather, it is the explicit justification for which values
are represented and which are not that is important.

A first step in evaluating the presentation of values in the research can be to determine if the approach is fundamentally descriptive or prescriptive. Prescriptive approaches advocate the primacy of particular values like egalitarian justice. Descriptive approaches simply reflect the values held by one or more stakeholder groups, with no pretensions that those values are the best. Both approaches have problems. If the approach to valuing is prescriptive, then one problem is that no single prescriptive value is agreed to be best. Moreover the nature of pluralistic interest-group democracy in the United States is such that pretensions about having the right set of values are not well received. Therefore, prescriptive theories should justify their particular prescriptions against other prescriptions and address the incompatibility of prescriptive ethics with the functioning of value pluralism in the United States. Descriptive approaches have different weaknesses and so need different safeguards. For example, since they usually draw their values from those held by some set of stakeholder groups, they need to justify the selection of particular stakeholder groups, given that limited time and resources usually preclude representing all such groups. Moreover, they should suggest whether and how to provide critical feedback to provide perspective on the descriptive values represented, because any particular group will be better or worse informed about the broader implications of their values.

Community researchers have discussed values as much or more than most researchers. In fact, a prescriptive stance on values is the hallmark of some major approaches to community research. Prescriptive values also enter community theories in other guises. For example, the choice to do research that supports those who are disenfranchised—certainly a central interest of the field—is often done in a way that is, in effect, an implicit endorsement of an egalitarian theory of justice. There are two potential problems with this kind of focus. One is that once the Pandora's box of prescriptive values is opened, it becomes increasingly difficult to justify the choice of one prescription over another. Why, for example, prefer egalitarian justice rather than libertarian justice? Why justice at all rather than human rights, equality, or liberty as prescriptive guides—especially since facilitating some of these values can conflict with others, as with the classic conflict between liberty and equality? Simply asserting that this is the value that one prefers is honest, but it does not help resolve the conflicts involved. Furthermore, such an approach flirts with an emotivist ethic, in which no ethic is better than another because all ethics are viewed as mere expressions of preference (MacIntyre, 1981). I prefer to see sensitivity to the range of prescriptive options we have, for they are far broader than most researchers recognize (Beauchamp, 1982).

The second potential problem with a prescriptive focus is that it is not clear that community researchers recognize the essential tension between such prescriptive values and the pluralism that drives political decision making in the United States. To oversimplify for the purpose of discussion, choosing to represent the disenfranchised may not win you friends at City Hall. Research cannot reflect the full diversity of values and interests that bear on a social problem when it takes a particular prescriptive position. This is a loss that should not be taken lightly in a field where social problem solving is valued so highly, and where social problem solving occurs primarily in the context of a pluralism of descriptive values. More careful attention in community research to broadly descriptive approaches to valuing might be beneficial, because such approaches would increase our ability to participate more effectively in the political process (Bryk, 1983; Scriven, 1980).

The descriptive approach strives to ensure that the values held by each group with a stake in a program or issue are represented. These values are used to help formulate research questions, identify preferred interventions and dependent variables, and interpret the results of the study. The notion of representing an array of values may run counter to some researchers' hope to be a voice for particular groups such as the disenfranchised. It is, nonetheless, in the interests of community researchers to consider the notion. For example, suppose the researcher is a political liberal whose interests in the disenfranchised lead toward research in social welfare policies and programs. Representing only liberal values in the research might lead to measuring such things as the amount of material needs provided to welfare recipients. However, this might not allow the researcher to answer the conservative's criticism that welfare policy increased dependence on the welfare system. In fact, this was exactly Murray's (1984) influential criticism of U.S. social welfare policy, and even social liberals found that they had to confront this issue if they wanted to participate fully in the relevant political debates.

Community research must be informed by and provide information about the entire array of relevant values if it is to be a full partner in the political process. No matter what one's own values are, designing one's research to take account of the strengths and weaknesses of values that differ from one's own is the surest way to avoid overlooking important arguments that bear on an issue. This is not an argument for a value-free science, but rather for explicit consideration of a plausible range of values, so that one's own values do not dominate the research and so limit its utility.

Constructing Knowledge

The fourth problem facing community researchers concerns our understanding of how scientists ought to construct knowledge. Therefore, one of the aspects of a theory of community research to be evaluated is how it handles both epistemological and methodological matters. When a theory tackles epistemological matters, it ought to try to go beyond the standard diatribe against logical positivism and to avoid egregious errors of fact about epistemological developments in the past 50 years—for example, by not saying that concepts like reality or causality have been rejected in modern epistemology, for both concepts are alive and well, albeit in substantially reconceptualized form (Humphreys, 1986; Leplin, 1984). It is fairer to convey accurately the breadth of opinion in modern epistemology, from classical epistemology through naturalized epistemology and social epistemology (Fuller, 1988) and to acknowledge that no one is generally viewed as having solved many of the trenchant problems like the nature of truth, the nature of scientific rationality, and the influence of rationality relative to the psychological and social causes of knowledge.

One rarely finds a social scientist with sufficient familiarity with the field to meet the criteria suggested by these problems, but a good example is Westergaard and Kelly's (1988) paper on the topic—a broad treatise with a fair and balanced view of these problems. If I part ways somewhat with those authors, it is because I see concepts like contextualism and conventionalism less as answers than as problems. They are just two among the multiple concepts that we can use to think about the problem of knowledge, and they have their own disadvantages. My own work on that topic places somewhat more emphasis on the value of generating a multiplicity of such concepts that give different perspectives on the problem of knowledge and appeals more to the role of self-reflection and social criticism as ongoing mechanisms for identifying the many biases that we can never eliminate from our work (Cook, 1986; Shadish, 1989).

These matters of epistemology blend into methodology at many points. Two examples are the issues of kinds of knowledge and characteristics of methods. The first issue, kinds of knowledge, refers to the fact that researchers can gather information about such diverse matters as the existence and magnitude of cause–effect relationships, mediating causal mechanisms, program implementation, client needs, generalizability, or construct validity. Our experimental heritage at first led us to think that questions of causal inference—does this program work?—were always most important. Today we know that other questions can be more important depending on the situation, so an important evaluative concern is the guidelines that a theory offers about how to choose questions for different situations.

The second issue, characteristics of methods, refers to the fact that no perfect method exists for answering any given question, so that a taxonomy of methodology is required that captures the multidimensional strengths and weaknesses of any given method. Excellence can be assessed by examining how well a theory addresses method choice, and in particular by how well it accounts for the diverse strengths and weaknesses of the methods that it recommends. For example, Cronbach (1982a) refers to a methodological trade-off between bandwidth versus fidelity. *Bandwidth* refers to the number of different kinds of questions that a method answers, and *fidelity* refers to the accuracy of the answer provided. Usually methods high in bandwidth, like the survey or the case study, are low in fidelity, and vice versa. To choose between methods high in bandwidth versus those high in fidelity, the researcher must decide how much reduction in uncertainty about each issue is tolerable in a given study (Shadish, 1986b). For some purposes, great certainty about the existence of a cause–effect relationship is needed—as when the question is whether a new drug causes a harmful side effect. But, other times, local citizens or federal policymakers are often quite willing to base actions on data that are less than certain, preferring pragmatism to scientific certainty. If, for example, decisions must be made quickly, if much high-quality knowledge is already available, or if little of importance hinges on a right or wrong answer relative to other questions also asked in the study (Berk & Rossi, 1977; Cronbach, 1982a), then the premium on fidelity may be smaller. A good theory helps make these and other methodological trade-offs clearer.

So when judging the merits of community research, it is important to consider these epistemological and methodological matters as well. Particular suspicion should be given to any claim to have the right answer in epistemology, or to any claim that any single methodology is the one that we should all be using most of the time. Conversely, highest regard should go to someone who uses a number of different ways to approach a problem when—as is most often the case—no single approach is uniformly the best, who thoughtfully acknowledges the strengths and weaknesses of each approach, and who works to ensure that the set of approaches used does not suffer from an overall constant bias of omission or commission (Shadish, 1989).

SUMMARY

In summary, then, when judging the merits of community research, I suggest asking four questions:

1. What is the implicit theory of social problem solving?
2. How could the resulting research be useful in social problem solving?
3. What values are implicated in the theory?
4. What approach to knowledge construction is advocated?

Of course, there are connections and overlaps among the questions so that one's answers to one question often imply answers to other questions. For example, the choice to pursue instrumental use tends to imply a local and incremental theory of social change. It is quite likely, therefore, that only a limited number of patterns of research practice could practically emerge from these assumptions—at least that is what my recent research about patterns of program evaluation practice implies (Shadish & Epstein, 1987).

THE THREE OTHER STEPS IN THE LOGIC OF EVALUATION

So far, all of this chapter has been concerned with the first step in the logic of evaluation—selection of criteria of merit. But the logic involves three more steps. Besides specifying criteria of merit, we must complete the second, third, and fourth steps if we want to judge the merits of community research. The second step of the logic is to set standards of performance for each criterion that say what level of performance on the criterion is sufficient to be called good. Those standards can take two forms: absolute and comparative. Absolute standards specify a level of performance that has to be achieved. Such standards are rare, but there are examples in methodological and statistical matters where some approaches are generally acknowledged to be superior for narrow purposes. For example, the structural modeling of latent variables improves on path analysis, in part because it copes better with problems of unreliability of measurement in the latter technique (Cook & Campbell, 1979). Another example of an absolute standard is my previous suggestion that any theory that discusses epistemology ought to avoid egregious errors of fact. In most cases, however, comparative standards are more practical and useful, where the thing being evaluated is compared with its competitors to evaluate relative performance on the criteria of merit. For example, not only does Westergaard and Kelly's (1988) discussion of epistemology meet the absolute standard of avoiding egregious errors of fact, it also fares well by the comparative standard that it is better reasoned and informed than many other epistemological discussions. We could also ask about other research specialties that are critical competitors to community research. For example, is community research doing a better job than program evaluation or policy analysis at solving the problems that we have in common? Answering this question is also part of judging the worth of community research.

The third step of the logic is to measure performance on the criteria. For the topic of community research, this is not something we are accustomed to do. An excellent example is the McClure et al. (1980) review, which suggested that most community research does not actualize basic community concepts such as intervening at a systems level. For each of us proposing criteria of merit in community research, therefore, we need to consider how we would assess whether community research lived up to our standards. To do so, we have to begin to think more specifically than the general prescriptions we have forwarded thus far.

Finally, the fourth step of the logic suggests that we synthesize the results of all our measurements into an overall value judgment about the worth of each thing we are evaluating. This step is difficult because, if we have more than one criteria of merit, as is nearly always the case, we have to develop some weighting scheme to combine results over criteria. The weighting scheme should reflect the differential importance that we assign to different criteria. In my own case, for example, I place somewhat less weight on ontological matters than on methodological matters, because assumptions about the latter seem more plausibly defended than assumptions about the former (e.g., whether there really is a reality). Whether right or wrong in the priorities assigned, such priorities are made explicit in the process of defending a weighting scheme. Such explication can only help improve the quality of our debates.

CONCLUSION

There was a time when many applied social researchers thought that they could judge the merits of community research using mostly methodological criteria. Our experimental heritage in psychology fostered this kind of thinking, and, in many ways, it served as well for years. With the benefit of several decades of field research experience, however, we now know that the criteria for good community research must be far broader than just methodological—although the methodological is still important. Such criteria must be broadly strategic in nature and invoke a host of issues about the role that community research should play in social problem solving, in value debates, in policy making, and in defining the nature of scientific knowledge. Such a broad approach is extraordinarily challenging because it forces us to consider criteria that go beyond our normal disciplinary training. Many other applied social research specialties face similar problems, which is no surprise, considering the extent to which they all share some aspirations to being agents of social problem solving. Perhaps we are all becoming part of a broader specialty of applied social research, each coming at the problem in the context of our individual historical context, but each butting heads with similar constraints. If so, then it behooves us to take these challenging criteria as seriously as possible to maximize the possibilities that community research will play at least as central and important a role in the next two decades as it has played in the past.

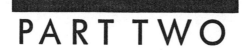

PART TWO

KEY CONCEPTS: FIVE APPROACHES TO FRAMING THE ENDEAVOR

CHAPTER 3

A CONTEXTUALIST EPISTEMOLOGY FOR ECOLOGICAL RESEARCH

CYNTHIA KINGRY-WESTERGAARD AND JAMES G. KELLY

We welcome the opportunity provided by this conference to examine the criteria for choosing between different methodologies and conceptual frameworks in Community Psychology. Psychologists, as well as philosophers of science, are now calling for a critical analysis of the theories and methods of empirical research in psychology (Altman & Rogoff, 1987; Ash & Woodward, 1988; Cronbach, 1986; McGuire, 1986; Meehl, 1986; Walsh, 1987a). For example, at a 1985 American Psychological Association symposium in celebration of the 1965 Swampscott Conference (Bennett, Anderson, Cooper, Hassol, Klein, & Rosenblum, 1966), Altman concluded that:

> Community psychology now needs to reflect on the philosophical issues that are central to any world view—units of analysis, time and change, and philosophy of science. By doing so, the field can enter its next stage of its life with a conscious understanding of its philosophical underpinnings. (1987, p. 627)

Making our philosophical assumptions explicit will facilitate the understanding of multifaceted phenomena in Community Psychology. Without explicit assumptions, researchers run the risk of tacitly endorsing assumptions that they themselves may not consider to be valid, authentic, apt, or robust for conducting research in Community Psychology.

In this chapter, we argue for an *Ecological* approach to community psychology. The guiding force of the Ecological approach is in its commitment to *Contextualism*. Contextualism is the epistemological theory that knowledge is relative to a given empirical and theoretical frame of reference and that we are implicitly embedded in the world we observe. Contextualism acknowledges the responsibility of the observer in choosing a given frame of reference and in justifying the chosen frame of reference. Contextualism requires that one be deliberately aware of the multifaceted nature of the conditions and motivations for the expression of behavior across environmental conditions. Contextualism also requires that observers be flexible in their selection of alternative or complementary methodologies when conducting research across different environmental conditions. Because of their commitment to the human responsibility of the construction of knowledge, contextualists are often called *constructivists* or *pragmatic realists* (Efran, Lukens, & Lukens, 1988; Giere, 1988). The Ecological approach advocates the use of alternative or complementary frameworks and methodologies when conducting community research. We hope to show that such an approach provides the most appropriate postpositivistic framework for characterizing the robust properties of community systems.

EPISTEMOLOGICAL THEORY AND METHODOLOGY: THE VALUE OF HAVING AN EXPLICIT EPISTEMOLOGY

It is now generally agreed, across a wide array of disciplines, that it is impossible to escape the implications of adopting a specific scientific method: The choice of method instructs us to record particular kinds of facts by using certain recognized procedures. Even if we are unaware of our own theoretical biases, we live with their effects. It is now recognized that

> . . . the nature of science in different periods has been determined by the methods employed in collecting facts and reasoning about them, and by the prevailing approach to the study of natural phenomena. (Hall, 1966, p. 159).

The history of philosophy of science contains many examples in which epistemological assumptions have affected the practice of science and shaped the evolution of human knowledge (Feyerabend, 1975, 1987; Giere, 1988; Gilligan, 1982; Hall, 1966; Hare-Mustin & Marecek, 1988; Keller, 1987; Lott, 1985; McGuire, 1986; Rose, 1987; Rosnow & Georgoudi, 1986; Suppe, 1974).

Epistemology is the analysis of the weighted importance of the observations, assumptions, and inferences that we make and of the justifications that we give for what we claim to know (Giere, 1988; Kornblith, 1985; Pappas & Swain, 1978; Quine & Ullian, 1970). More often than not, however, scientific disciplines have functioned with only an implicit knowledge of their epistemological assumptions. This has often had the consequence of generating "scientific paradigms" that contain principles or assumptions with which many researchers would disagree, if those principles or assumptions were made explicit. It also creates a narrowly focused worldview, or way of doing science, which precludes consideration of alternative metaphysical or epistemological assumptions in the practice of a given field of research.

The importance of epistemological techniques and assumptions, implicit or explicit, is not a concern that is specific to or even arises only out of community psychology inquiry. Contextualist epistemologies have emerged forcefully in several disciplines. Two examples are presented from the biological and psychological sciences. A further contribution comes from feminist epistemology.

CONTEXTUALISM IN BIOLOGY AND PSYCHOLOGY

Kauffman (1971) and Wimsatt (1974) have independently argued for an explanatory model in the biological sciences that consists of a multivariate, multidimensional analysis of a given system. Kauffman and Wimsatt argue that there are multiple frames of reference for the observation of a given system (or subsystem) and that there is no preferred method. The researcher's role is to delineate the boundaries of his or her frame of reference, given personal interests, questions, and concepts of what is relevant to the research. Within such boundaries, certain things are "knowable," and some are inaccessible or excluded.

Kauffman (1971) showed that "an organism may be seen as doing indefinitely many things, and may be decomposed into parts and processes in indefinitely many ways." Then, given a chosen description of the organism as doing some particular thing, "we will use that description to help us decompose the organism into particular parts and processes which articulate together to cause it to behave as described." Kauffman argued that the descriptions of parts and processes of an organism from one theoretical or methodological frame of reference "need only be compatible with, and not deducible from, the descriptions of parts and processes articulated by a different decomposition" (Kauffman, 1971, pp. 258–259). His decompositional analysis allows the researcher to self-consciously choose the boundaries that frame what is to be observed or investigated in a specific context.

Kauffman and Wimsatt argue that examining the integration and interconnections of the many functional parts of a given system can provide the researcher with a more robust and ecologically valid interpretation or representation of an individual and the system(s) within which the person is embedded (Kauffman, 1971; Wimsatt, 1974, 1981). According to Wimsatt, "robustness" measures the reliability of the theories and methods of science. Because we have no absolute or a priori criteria with which to validate our theories, models, observations, or values, we must check them against each other. In doing so, we discover contradictions in the assumptions and techniques that produce them.

The Ecological approach to Community Psychology shares Wimsatt's belief in the "robustness" of human knowledge that does not appeal to the "fixed" or "objective" properties of objects themselves to distinguish knowledge from illusion or false belief. Instead, the Ecological approach relies on the logical and empirical coherence of the information obtained by multiple methods and observations, each considered in context. "Robustness" in terms of the Ecological approach implies an analysis of the discriminant and convergent validity of concepts.

Consistent with the contextualist and multivariate, multilevel, and systemic analysis of the Ecological approach, Shadish (1986a) argues that *critical multiplism* will enhance research in psychology. Critical multiplism acknowledges the unique set of biases associated with a given research design or analysis. It acknowledges that no single approach provides the true characterization of a system and that researchers are "constantly engaged in a battle against the partial validity of the methods that are available" (Shadish, Cook, & Houts, 1986, p. 43). Multiple methods and analyses complement each other, compensating for the limitations of each other, to contribute convergent and discriminant validity of our claims to knowledge (Shadish et al., 1986). Planned critical multiplism provides "tools to help scientists explore the boundaries of their knowledge" (Shadish et al., 1986, p. 43), that is, to help them identify the specific assumptions, methods, values, and biases which constrain research and which produce claims to knowledge (Shadish, 1986a).

Congruent with these Contextualist analyses, many feminists are also reevaluating the validity of claims to knowledge made from a positivistic, value- or observer-free perspective.

CONSTRUCTIVISM AND CONTEXTUALISM IN FEMINIST EPISTEMOLOGY

The contributions of a feminist epistemology, although complementary to those of Kauffman and Wimsatt, differ in that they advocate the recognition, authenticity, and importance of a distinctly female point of view, a distinctly female sociopolitical unit (structure, construct) in a community setting, and the structural and functional roles defined for those units (Flax, 1983; Gilligan, 1982; Harding, 1987; Harding & O'Barr, 1987; Hare-Mustin & Marecek, 1988; Harstock, 1983; Hoffman, 1981; Keller, 1983, 1987; Lott, 1985; Luepnitz, 1988a, 1988b; McVicker-Clinchy & Belenky, 1987; Riger, this volume; Wallston, 1981; M. R. Walsh, 1987).

For example, Belenky, McVicker-Clinchy, Goldberger, and Tarule (1986) saw that this feminist constructivist viewpoint had important implications for epistemology. First, the women they interviewed in their work were not just considered "subjects," but "key, active participants" who felt "empowered" by being understood and represented. Second, the need to develop a capacity to listen beyond traditional interviewing techniques was understood and appreciated. Third, according to McVicker-Clinchy and Belenky (1987), connected knowers are not dispassionate unbiased observers. Connected knowers try to see the phenomena examined from another point of view. The epistemology of the connected knower focuses on data not just as evidence to support a given hypothesis but as a guide to the experiences of the knower (McVicker-Clinchy & Belenky, 1987, p. 12). Feminists have shown that there is flexibility in our choice of "units of analysis" in a given system or setting; hence, they too are committed to a constructivist or contextualist theory of knowledge.

From a contextualist perspective, the choice of research methods is greatly influenced by the interests, values, and assumptions of the researcher (Belenky, et al., 1986; Falicov, 1988; Fish, 1983; Gilligan, 1982; Harding, 1987; Harding & Hintikka, 1983; Hare-Mustin & Marecek, 1988; Lott, 1985; McVicker-Clinchy & Belenky, 1987; Parlee, 1981; Ruback & Innes, 1988; Wallston, 1981). The assumptions of an Ecological Contextualist approach create interests and activities that diverge from traditional, positivistic research models.

A CONTEXTUALIST EPISTEMOLOGY FOR ECOLOGICAL RESEARCH IN COMMUNITY PSYCHOLOGY

The topic of ecology has had several key proponents who have helped shape and define a contextualist understanding of behavior. The works of Roger Barker and colleagues (Barker, 1960, 1968, 1987a, 1987b), Gregory Bateson (Bateson, 1972; also Luepnitz, 1988a), and Urie Bronfenbrenner (Bronfenbrenner, 1977, 1979, 1986; also Falicov, 1988) stand out in particular. The ecological approach of Bateson and colleagues has emphasized the various levels and types of communities in community research (Kelly, 1966, 1968, 1979a, 1979b, 1986b, 1987; Kelly, Dassoff, Levin, Schreckengost, Stelzner, & Altman, 1988; Kelly & Hess, 1987; Kelly, Ryan, & Altman, in press; Trickett, 1984; Trickett & Birman, 1988; Trickett, Kelly, & Todd, 1972; Trickett, Kelly, & Vincent, 1985; Trickett & Mitchell, in press; Vincent & Trickett, 1983).

The Ecological approach defines the relationship between the observer and the observed (participant) as the source for the construction of meaning about the phenomena to be studied. Thus, persons and systems become understandable when they are considered a part of a multilevel, multistructured, multidetermined social context. Moreover, persons and systems may appear less tangible in virtue of the multifaceted ways in which their boundaries and complexity can be articulated.

The Ecological approach affirms that it is not possible to understand the meaning of persons or systems in context unless the observer and persons to be observed develop mutual criteria for their definition of *context*. The various multiple features of the context are considered to affect both the observer and participants. Both are considered to be part of the particular context where observations take place. The relationship between the observer (scientist or researcher) and the observed (participant) itself becomes a topic of research. A further definition of the process of understanding phenomena is that the observer is dependent on the creation of a reciprocal working relationship with the persons(s) or system(s) observed, not only to select a preferred topic for research, but also to define their own working relationship. Four facets can be identified as constituting the Ecological approach.

Facet One: Theoretical Propositions

Ten theoretical propositions affect the expression of constraints and resources in contexts and characterize the interrelationships of persons and settings:

1. Concepts about persons and settings are derived from the observer and participants appreciating their own contexts and constructing a mutual understanding of their shared context.
2. Persons in context are observed in terms of their role performance in creating resources and coping with personal, organizational, and community constraints.
3. Social settings are observed in terms of the operation of social norms as they affect the definition, use, and response to resources and constraints.
4. Social settings define the shared meaning and experience of persons and include being a member of a context where occasions, places, and events define and maintain social norms.
5. Adaptive behavior is defined in terms of the resources that persons and settings create, use, maintain, and replenish.
6. Adaptive behavior and the criteria for adaptive behavior may vary from place to place, and from time to time.
7. Relationships are reciprocal: Persons affect settings, and settings affect persons; persons influence other persons, and one setting affects another setting.
8. Events, settings, and persons outside the immediate social setting affect the expression of structures, roles, and norms inside social settings.
9. Person–setting transactions in one setting indirectly produce tangible effects for the interactions of other persons in other settings.
10. Social processes can facilitate or inhibit the interdependence of persons and social settings and the interdependence of roles and social norms.

Facet Two: The Social Construction of Ecological Knowledge

The ecological approach focuses on the behavior of persons in social settings related to the social construction that the participants, both observer and observed, create of their own context. It is assumed that different participants may create different constructions of their context. Observations are bound by space, time, and the histories of role relationships of the participants.

What becomes essential in the elaboration of the Ecological approach is that the participants are able to consciously articulate the unique constraints and opportunities that affect their own context. A requirement for initiating a construction of their own context is that the researcher and participants must invest themselves in the ambiguity of the discovery process. Whatever understanding of phenomena is developed has an explicit bounded quality that communicates and denotes the nature of the observations in their sociopolitical, spatiotemporal context.

What is theoretically construed about persons and social settings comes about as the researcher learns about and experiences the events and processes related to the social construction of his or her contexts and the context(s) of the participants. The social construction of context frames the observations about roles, norms, and their interdependence in social settings.

According to this Ecological approach, theoretical propositions are tested, measured, and understood by the meaning that the propositions have for the participants who are experiencing the phenomenon. Understanding the expression of social roles and social norms requires that the participants develop a process and a plan to be informed about each other's community or system of study, and about their own working context.

Facet Three: The Collaborative Style

Under the ecological approach, the style of work is collaborative among the participants. The process of collaborative work involves both the researcher and the other participants defining a working relationship for the integration of research and practice. The researcher and other participants are expected to appreciate the value of their work together in redefining the research activity. The collaborative style reaffirms that research hypotheses are derived from the collaboration of the participants in the context of their working relationship. This working relationship focuses on a shared understanding of the operation of social structures, roles, and norms as they occur in given contexts. The assumed benefit of the collaborative style is that the discovery of information about the structures, roles, and norms expressed in context will enhance the authenticity, the validity, and, therefore, the usefulness of the research.

The epistemological significance of the collaborative relationship is that it occurs in a context in which ideas are tested, elaborated, redefined, examined, reexamined, and evolved. The collaborative relationship becomes a social structure by which the processes of discovery and understanding can take place. The observer (researcher) and the observed (participants), in this relationship, then create together a shared agenda to discover and to understand community contexts.

Facet Four: Social Processes

The validity of Ecological research is realized only if the participants understand their context or agenda-specific interests and roles in the collaborative enterprise. Understanding the processes of collaboration and the stages and sequences involved in the design of research and interventions is necessary for creating contextual knowledge.

This facet is concerned with how techniques and methods are interdependent with settings. Social settings become meaningful because of the sequences of social interactions that they set in motion. The study of social processes makes it possible to understand how roles and social norms create social structures, how social structures make roles and norms interdependent with persons and settings, and the processes of constructing knowledge. The ecological approach gives attention to the sequence of stages, steps, and activities that gives unique meaning to any particular social context.

IMPLICATIONS OF A CONTEXTUALIST, ECOLOGICAL EPISTEMOLOGY

The Ecological approach emphasizes a sequence of activities in which the researcher understands, learns, and becomes informed about phenomena in context. The researcher is prepared to develop and to revise his or her concepts as the collaborative relationship evolves. What is not consistent with the Ecological approach is for the researcher to recruit or to persuade the participants to help test out concepts or hypotheses that are developed or selected solely by the researcher. In that case, the researcher is denying or not attending to the participants' own context. Research activity according to the Ecological approach is inductive, exploratory, improvisational, and requires constant testing and feedback; testing of ideas occurs by going back and forth between the concepts and the experience of the researcher and the participants. These activities must all take place before the official, public, or "real" research or intervention(s) can begin.

The four facets of the Ecological approach are interdependent; as each facet is addressed, meaning is given to each of the other facets and to the total context. Appreciating context allows the researcher to listen to the voices of others and provides the opportunity for understanding and empowering others. For both researcher and participants, "gaining a voice" presupposes dialogue, networking, and empathic listening and intervention. The ecological approach also acknowledges that the research process is constructed and influenced by its spatiotemporal and sociopolitical parameters, agendas, or frames of reference (Fish, 1983; Hare-Mustin & Maracek, 1988; Katz & Kahn, 1978; Kelly, Altman, Kahn, Stokols, & Rausch, 1986; Lott, 1985; Parlee, 1981; Ruback & Innes, 1988).

The Ecological approach adapts research styles to incorporate initial uncertainty and ambiguity as the collaborative enterprise is initiated. In this sense, research becomes an "open" process, because there is tolerance for checking the validity of assumptions, the efficacy of actions, and the very definition and meaning of research. The Ecological approach is empiricist, exploratory, collaborative, and contextual in its theoretical and methodological assumptions. Research that is ecological can provide an opportunity to understand what is complex and unique about a given setting or context.

CONCLUSION

It is our view that research performed under the philosophical assumptions and methodologies of Positivism has had the effect of reducing our knowledge about the complex and unique constraints and qualities of a given "system" and that such a research style is outside the aspirations of the field of Community Psychology. We propose that a contextualist, Ecological epistemology provides the freedom to pursue lines of inquiry more congruent with the philosophical and sociopolitical interests of Community Psychology.

In this chapter we have argued that an Ecological approach may provide a useful theoretical framework for the development of research strategies in Community Psychology. Our aim has been to show the value of alternative points of view and alternative investigative techniques. We believe such an approach is more congruent, compatible, and logically consistent with the aims and aspirations of the field of Community Psychology.

In closing, we recall Cronbach's comments, made in response to a 1983 conference on the potentialities for knowledge in social science. This chapter has been written with a feeling of intellectual kinship and the shared spirit of Cronbach's affirmations:

> The style and procedures preferred for one inquiry can be ill-suited for another topic or at another stage in the evolution of knowledge or for an investigator in different circumstances. With that caveat, I recapitulate a few preferences I have suggested: for more exploratory work, for less emphasis on the magnitude and statistical significance of "effect sizes," for more effort to record concomitant and intermediate events that help explain local variation, for more discussion of research plans and interpretations with peers having disparate backgrounds. Each piece of research should be an effort to give an unimpeachable and reasonably full account of events in a time, place, and context. Multiple interpretations of information already in hand will often be more instructive, at less cost, than additional data gathering. I have encouraged critical analysis of research methods and their further development, along with substantive criticism of extrapolations. To advocate pluralistic tolerance of alternative accounts is in no way to advocate tender-mindedness.[1]

---

[1]From the chapter "Social Inquiry by and for Earthlings" in *Metatheory in Social Science: Pluralisms and Subjectives*, edited by D. W. Fiske and R. A. Shweder. Copyright 1986, University of Chicago Press. Reprinted with permission.

CHAPTER 4

DEVELOPMENTAL ANALYSES OF COMMUNITY PHENOMENA

RAYMOND P. LORION

As the discipline of community psychology enters its third decade, the breadth of its agenda and the complexity of its methodological challenges are becoming increasingly understood. Central to both is the need to examine, monitor, and control processes related to change. The uniqueness of our discipline lies in its concern with change as it occurs at and through the interface between the individual and the environment. As I will explain later, attending to processes of change inevitably forces us to emphasize the temporal nature of the phenomena that we study. That focus involves the discipline in developmental inquiry. The intent of this chapter is to examine some of the implications of that inquiry for the discipline's evolution.

The importance of understanding change is not unique to our discipline. By definition, that focus is an element of all science. What is unique, however, is that the change processes of concern to community psychology are those reflecting individuals in interaction with the psychosocial and environmental systems within which they live. Consequently, we are confronted with the need to understand change as it occurs in individuals, in systems, and, most important, in their interaction.

The centrality of the study of change to scientific inquiry is clearly explained by Nunnally (1982):

> . . . most scientific theories and related research activities are concerned
> with some form of natural or experimentally induced change. This is evi-
> dent in research on the "big bang" theory of the origin of the universe,
> natural selection in the evolution of animal species, and the growth-and-
> decline prototheory that guides much of the research on human development
> and eventual aging. . . . Of course the effort in all experiments is to induce

changes, in a neat and orderly way, rather than sift through observations of natural changes that might provide circumstantial evidence with respect to a hypothesis. (p. 133)

By definition, change occurs over time. Consequently, its study requires methodologies that monitor the temporal processes of the phenomena under study.

THE TEMPORAL DIMENSION

As noted, seeking to understand the nature of change and the mechanisms by which phenomena are altered in form or extent places us squarely within the realm of developmental inquiry. Time becomes a main effect in our research designs. For individuals, this dimension may be defined in terms of weeks, months, or years, in terms of subjects' chronological age or achievement of developmental milestones, or in terms of maturational sequences. Community psychology's challenge is to establish comparable developmental indices to differentiate the maturational stage of the programs and organizations that it studies. It must create a taxonomy for differentiating the evolutionary status of relevant transactional processes. The discipline will thereby become able to examine systematically the evolutionary mechanisms that underlie person–environment interactions.

Toward that goal, we have much to learn from our developmental colleagues. Developmental researchers, for example, approach the study of time using three principal strategies. The first, the cross-sectional design, provides insight into time-related phenomena by simultaneously sampling at selected points along the temporal dimension. Depending on their extent, direction, and consistency, group differences are interpreted as inferential evidence of an underlying developmental process.

Lorion, Cowen, and Caldwell (1975), for example, used this design to examine the construct validity of a teacher rating scale for assessing classroom adjustment in primary-grade children. By comparing the behavioral profiles of children across academic-year levels, the investigators were able to determine the measure's sensitivity to expected developmental patterns. Similarly, Tolan (1987) used a cross-sectional design to obtain preliminary confirmation of a hypothesized link between the completion of adolescent developmental tasks and involvement in antisocial and delinquent behavior. Documentation of that link cross-sectionally provided the evidence needed to justify the design and conduct of research to replicate the finding in a prospective, longitudinal study.

Only through the conduct of prospective research can one validate the existence of developmental processes and uncover the mechanisms through which they occur. Such research requires the adoption of a within-subjects design and the planful monitoring of the phenomena of concern through the use of multiple measurement probes. Such studies, however, are costly in terms of time and resources. To date, most have paid limited attention to the ongoing contribution of environmental factors. Undoubtedly, the continuous monitoring of ecological elements represents a major challenge for community psychology. Yet, without prospective data, it is not possible to confirm operative developmental processes and, for our purposes, to design interventions that consistently result in desired changes.

The challenge of such research is that it is the captive of "real time." To study processes that evolve over a decade or more, one must conduct investigations lasting at least that long. The necessary planning, piloting, and data-analytic stages may double the actual time required to conduct such research. For that reason, the use of a multiple sequential cohort design often serves as an intermediate step between a cross-sectional and longitudinal study. The multiple cohorts are composed of samples at various stages along the relevant developmental continuum. Their inclusion in the study provides some of the time-saving advantages of the cross-sectional approach. The inclusion of sequential measurement allows for the identification and monitoring of operative processes. If carefully planned, such designs can provide heuristically valuable approximations of the nature and consequence of the developmental mechanisms to be studied. Such approximations may be sufficient to design interventions to alter such mechanisms. If not, they can certainly inform one of what to consider in a longitudinal analysis.

Typically, these three designs have been applied in the study of individuals. They are, however, also applicable to the study of community groups and organizational systems. An important first step would be to establish a continuum along which the maturity of such entities can be differentiated. Sarason (1972) provided the discipline with a framework for conceptualizing the evolution of an organization. We must now translate that framework into psychometrically sound assessment procedures.

CHARACTERISTICS OF DEVELOPMENTAL RESEARCH

The incorporation of time within one's research design is a necessary but not entirely sufficient element for the conduct of developmental research, whether focused on behavior or on community phenomena. Santostefano (1978) and, more recently, Sroufe and Rutter (1984) have identified "a number of agreed-upon propositions that underlie all major developmental perspectives" (Sroufe & Rutter, 1984, p. 20). Their relevance to our discipline is important. Their adoption by the discipline will require creativity and systematic methodological research. Justifying that effort is their potential for expanding our knowledge base. They are as follows:

1. *Holism.* The meaning of a phenomenon cannot be determined independent of the context in which it occurs. As discussed below, this element is central to the transactional framework that postulates a reciprocal relationship between the individual and the environment, whereby each affects the nature of the other through a continuous synergistic process. By extension, one cannot understand an organization independent of its sociocultural context or a classroom independent of the school and the neighborhood in which it exists.

2. *Directedness.* From this perspective, events do not occur randomly. Rather, they are determined by a combination of individual and contextual characteristics that are based on both current and past experiences. As Sroufe and Rutter (1984) state:

> Later experience is not a random influence on individuals because persons selectively perceive, respond to, and create experience based on all that has gone on before. A child that isolates himself is not experiencing the same nursery school class as the child who engages other children. Also relevant here is the idea that development does not occur as a series of linear additions. Rather, development is characterized by reorganization of both old and new elements. Thus, reorganized, even previously existing elements are transformed. The "same" behavior may have totally new meaning with development, just as it may have different meanings in different contexts. (p. 20)

This same appreciation of the evolutionary nature of change across time and situation can be applied to our study of community entities and processes. Thus, for example, we can begin to look at a subgroup's place within the larger community as reflective of a series of prior interactions between each of these units.

3. *Differentiation of means and goals.* Over time, individuals gain access to an increasing array of ways to respond to situations and cope with adaptive demands. Through this process, they gain flexibility in how they will and can respond to an event. These alternatives become organized in ways that result in both predictability and diversity in response patterns. An understanding of these organizational patterns provides insight into both inter- and intraindividual differences. Thus, a variety of responses become alternative "means" to a particular "goal"; the meaning of each response must therefore be assessed in relation to its intended goal or outcome. This principle can also be extended beyond the level of the individual. What is posited is that community entities also evolve in complexity and response range. They also gain flexibility in the face of challenges to the achievement of their goals and the continuation of their survival. Presumably, it is possible to identify considerable variation in how communities pursue specific purposes. Therefore, we will learn to examine a community's behavior, at least in part, in terms of its intended outcomes. Understanding how communities link "means" and "ends" and the circumstances that inhibit or facilitate this process will contribute importantly to our discipline's ability to understand the creation of optimally humanizing settings.

4. *Mobility of behavioral functions.* As noted, increases in the range and diversity of responses to situations occur with time. Prior responses evolve in complexity and effectiveness. Through this process, the individual gains an increasing armamentarium of strategies for resolving adaptive demands. The principle of mobility refers to the fact that the array of alternatives is available and may be used in times of demand. It also posits that complex and evolved approaches may be set aside for the simple strategies characteristic of prior

stages. As Sroufe and Rutter (1984) note, maladaptation results from the inflexible use of previous modes of functioning in response rather than their use per se.

5. *The problems of continuity and change.* "The central proposition underlying a developmental perspective is that the course of development is lawful" (Sroufe & Rutter, 1984, p. 21). Unquestionably, as change occurs over time in the individual, group, organization, or community, significant qualitative differences will occur in the nature and extent of its "strategies" for responding to demands. Nevertheless, it is assumed that there is a continuity between early and late performance and early and late policies and programs. Underlying such change is a coherence that reflects the operation of identifiable, measurable, and, theoretically at least, controllable lawful processes. Clarification of the coherence and sequence of the pertinent processes represents a fundamental goal of developmental inquiry in community psychology.

Thus, in addition to the incorporation of time within one's experimental design, the developmental perspective assumes that behavior can best be understood as synergistically determined along the dimension of time, directed, lawful, ecologically appropriate, and coherent. Because of this coherence, it is possible to identify precursors to current states and, presumably, future pathways.

In thinking about applying developmental principles to our discipline's research, it may be helpful to delineate specifically what we perceive as the bounds that distinguish our discipline from such related fields as environmental psychology, clinical psychology, clinical child psychology, developmental psychopathology, and health psychology. I would propose that our distinctiveness lies in community psychology's concern with understanding emotional and behavioral health and dysfunction as it appears within people who exist within physical, psychosocial and political settings.

To achieve this perspective, the discipline has adopted an ecological perspective, wherein behavior's adaptive meaning is determined in terms of the individual within context. Thus, the individual and the context represent a single conceptual unit. As I will explain shortly, the transactional model offered by developmental theorists represents a valuable heuristic for understanding how emotional and behavioral states evolve, can be predicted and can be altered. Within that model, the synergistic or recurrent transactions occurring between individual and environmental factors are emphasized. I would propose that our discipline's defining focus is on the study of the transactions underlying development and their prediction and ultimate control.

A TRANSACTIONAL MODEL OF PREVENTIVE INTERVENTION RESEARCH

As I have explained elsewhere (Lorion, 1983, 1987; Lorion & Allen, 1989; Lorion, Price, & Eaton, 1988), preventive intervention research provides an excellent illustration of how a developmental framework extends our discipline's scientific rigor. The transactional model, for example, allows for the following definition of preventive intervention research:

> Prevention research can be conceptualized as applied developmental analyses involving the identification and systematic manipulation of processes related to the development of adaptive/maladaptive behavioral constellations in order to increase or decrease respectively the rate or level at which those behavioral constellations occur in the general population or some part thereof.

This definition highlights my belief that the design of preventive interventions should be based on knowledge of the processes underlying the transition of risk factors and precursor conditions to emotional and behavioral impairment. This definition imposes heavy demands on the preventive intervention researcher. It assumes that psychometrically sound procedures must be developed to distinguish the presence and absence of the outcome. It assumes that risk factors and precursor conditions can be identified and independently validated. It assumes that the necessary preintervention research has been conducted to develop psychometrically sound procedures for assessing risk in individuals or subgroups and for monitoring the implementation and impact of the intervention over time. Most important, however, it assumes the existence of a temporal model of the disorder's etiology.

To meet that challenge, we must obtain information on when and how "onset" of the target of concern occurs (e.g., Is it a sudden or prolonged process? Does it reflect a singular event or a sequential series of increasingly problematic states?), the nature and timing of its evolutionary process (e.g., How long is it from onset to the presentation of diagnostic signs?), and the anticipated "half-life" (i.e., the duration) of the intervention's effectiveness. The complexity of each of these temporal issues increases as one's focus shifts from individuals to organizations and communities. By what criteria, for example, does one define the "beginning" of an organizational or community "problem?" (Indeed, of a community!) The temporal elements of the model called for should inform one about when to initiate the intervention, how long it should last, at what points "booster" sessions may be needed, and when to assess effectiveness.

As stated, Sameroff's (Sameroff & Chandler, 1975; Sameroff & Fiese, 1988) "transactional perspective" offers a heuristically valuable framework within which to pose and to organize the aforementioned temporal questions. It simultaneously highlights the need to look beyond the individual to the environment to understand the former and back to the individual to understand the latter. It underlines the necessity of temporal concern, the pursuit of lawful connections between the elements of an ecological perspective, and the assumption that there is a coherence to the evolution of human functioning.

Sameroff's model evolved out of the struggle to confirm prospectively the causes of early childhood dysfunction suggested through retrospective analyses. Repeatedly, prospective examination of individual early risk factors did not result in their confirmation. At the same time, infants without such risks subsequently developed disorders. Careful examination of the histories of numerous cases of childhood disorder revealed that a second dimension also needed to be considered, that is, the receptivity and support of the environment within which the child is nurtured.

Importantly, Sameroff and his colleagues found that the accurate prediction of risk required not merely the simultaneous consideration of both individual and environmental dimensions but also recognition that the dimensions have a "transactional" relationship. Each affects the other through a continuous synergistic process. In effect, the model implies that "risk" results from the simultaneous presence of individual and environmental characteristics that influence each other in specifiable ways.

This sequence of mutual, reciprocal influence defines the developmental trajectory that, if unaltered, leads to dysfunction and distress. Schematically, the model would be reflected in a helical pattern in which individual and environmental factors continuously connect. Such interactions are the points at which mutual influences are exchanged and the transformed factors create the circumstances for their subsequent reconnection. Presumably, this process occurs continuously over time. One would speculate that "critical periods" exist in which the speed of the process and the "influenceability" of each factor vary in behaviorally meaningful ways.

The discipline needs to encourage research that elucidates how significant community-based organizations evolve over time. At issue is whether the aforementioned continuum of organizational stages can be described in heuristically meaningful ways. In his analysis of how social settings evolve, Sarason (1972) provides a framework for such research. He notes, for example, that to understand an organization or program, one needs to clarify the history of the decisions preceding its beginning. He also notes that the enthusiasm of program developers frequently needs to be recreated to sustain program effectiveness. Such factors may both inform one of program goals and provide an index of program momentum. Potentially, these elements will enhance our ability to define systemic stages.

APPLYING THE MODEL TO CURRENT RESEARCH

If correct, Sameroff's model of development significantly complicates prevention research's generative task. We must now simultaneously monitor individual and environmental processes. Justification for this added complexity is found in the unsatisfactory levels of predictive accuracy typically reported for either child or adult dysfunction. The inadequacy of considering only individual variables, for example, is suggested by data that we are currently analyzing from the Knoxville Basic Academic Skills Enhancement (BASE) project (Lorion, Hightower, Work, & Shockley, 1987; Lorion, Work, & Hightower, 1984). We now have five-year prospective follow-up data with which to assess the predictive accuracy of our risk-identification procedures. The challenge confronting us is to determine which set of factors to attend to in assessing individual risk. Indeed, we need to consider that this assessment may not be made reliably for individuals but only for sub-groups, that is, only in terms of the individual–situation units described earlier.

This possibility arises when one considers one of the project's initial findings. We discovered that children with remarkably comparable profiles of academic readiness and developmental maturity display quite different levels of basic academic skills by the end of their first year of school. Both the classroom and the particular school building within which their original abilities and potential were to develop had important consequences for the children's academic progress.

We find that within the classroom we need to consider not only the teacher's experience and expectations, but also the variation in potential among the peer group. Thus, we need to understand how the classroom environment both influences and reflects the abilities and potential of individual children. In turn, we need to develop strategies for modeling how students and the classroom synergistically alter each other. It may be, for example, that specific patterns of variation in student readiness promote maximal individual development, whereas other variations inhibit the optimal acquisition of basic academic skills. Patterns of student groupings may increase or decrease a teacher's capacity to instruct, to maintain discipline, and to enjoy the setting.

Understanding developmental processes that we wish to modify from the transactional perspective requires that we abandon the simplistic assumption that prior states or abilities provide direct access to information about future events. Rather, we need to understand that prior states alter and are altered by host situations in complex ways. In our research, for example, we sought to understand the contribution of teacher assumptions about children from disadvantaged families to the children's academic progress (Neimann, 1987). We learned that such attitudes depend both on the teacher's underlying attitudes and immediate experience with specific parents. In turn, parental views toward education and willingness to communicate with teachers depended on the parents' assumptions about the teacher's views, which reciprocally reflected the teacher's assumptions about the parents.

In analyzing our data, we must recognize the reactivity of the BASE project. From the outset, it became apparent that ours was not an unobtrusive study. During the pilot trial of the screening program, word-of-mouth reports of our presence apparently increased preregistration of kindergarten children to record levels. As a nascent intervention, we affected the school's ecology in ways that we have yet to understand. We need to learn more about the particular mix of teachers who chose to participate. Their assumptions about the career implications of program involvement and their expectations regarding the community's acceptance of the program presumably influenced our outcomes. Similar questions can be raised about the families who chose to participate in our "experiment."

At this point, however, our research is just beginning to exploit the potential of the Sameroff model. Our challenge is how to monitor the "transaction" and, thereby, accurately predict how a child's makeup shapes and is shaped by the physical and social environment within which the child lives and learns. To do so, we must infer and test models of relevant transactional processes.

We are also beginning a series of studies on the initiation of substance involvement in preadolescent and adolescent children, which we hope will further test the Sameroff model. Our reviews of available knowledge have enabled us to identify both individual and environmental variables that are relevant to predicting risk for substance abuse (Lorion, Bussell, & Goldberg, in press). We believe that we can identify elements consistent with Sameroff's "continuum of reproductive risk" (i.e., individual constitutional risks) and with the "continuum of caretaking casualty" (i.e., relevant environmental risks). We have yet, however, to find a clear specification of how each influences the state of the other. We are also concerned that environmental risks may require the specification of a "continuum of peer influence" and a "continuum of familial influence" as well as the delineation of other elements of the child's ecology.

For example, we are beginning to work with a model for predicting a child's "intent to use." We are speculating that among the elements that we must consider to make that prediction are the child's knowledge of and attitudes toward substance use, the child's calculation of the relative merits and costs of use, the child's assumptions about peer use and acceptance of use, and the child's access to substances and opportunities for their use. These elements are part of the peer environment. Yet, according to the model, we must also consider the child's family environment. Examples of variables that we believe must be examined are parental and sibling attitudes toward substance use, the degree of attention that is paid to the child's emotional and behavioral state, and the family's level of substance involvement.

As stated, however, this array of variables must be considered in ways other than traditional linear analyses. In effect, we must produce prospective evidence that individual elements alter environmental elements, which, in turn, produce identifiable changes in individual elements, and so forth. It is this sequential analysis that distinguishes transactional from simple multivariate explanations of behavior. Whereas the former is dynamic, the latter is static. We believe that the Piagetian concepts of assimilation and accommodation (Piaget, 1952) apply to understanding evolution of the decision to initiate, continue, and cease substance involvement. The methodological challenge confronting us is to monitor the transactions of person and environment that define that decisional process. The complexity of this empirical task is well described by Sarason and Doris (1979):

> From the transactional perspective, heredity and environment are never dichotomous. It can even be misleading to say they "interact" because that is more often than not interpreted in terms of effects of heredity on environment just as for so long we have paid attention to the effects of parents on children and virtually ignored the influence of children on parents. The transactional approach is always a two-way street. (p. 25)

Monitoring such processes will require new methodologies and innovative solutions to long-standing problems. For example, the continuous monitoring of substance-related knowledge, attitudes, and behaviors is likely to be highly reactive. Attributing directionality to observed relationships between individual changes and environmental changes will require the use of very large samples and, in all likelihood, the incorporation of multiple replications within the same data collection format. The goal in such research would be both to validate the transactional model and, more important, to develop the knowledge base required to design effective strategies for the prevention of substance-related disorders.

APPLICATION OF THE DEVELOPMENTAL APPROACH TO OTHER COMMUNITY ISSUES

In his presidential address to the American Psychological Association's Division of Community Psychology, Heller (1988) challenged us to link our rhetoric about community with our research. As he noted, for the most part we remain focused on the study of individuals. "Community" for many of us represents the location of our research rather than its focus. Heller proposes that we need to shift our focus so that "community-as-setting" and "community-as-feeling" become central to the questions that we ask and the interventions that we propose.

I expect that such research would need to be firmly rooted within the developmental perspective described herein. I assume that we will discover that both concepts of community have important temporal dimensions, are directed, lawful and coherent, and proceed through a series of evolving stages. I would also assume that communities per se are involved in a transactional relationship with the broader social and cultural context. If so, our discipline again is challenged to focus its attention on the transactional nexus between factors that influence human functioning. The study of such processes would unquestionably represent an enriching focus for our discipline.

CHAPTER 5

WAYS OF KNOWING AND ORGANIZATIONAL APPROACHES TO COMMUNITY RESEARCH

STEPHANIE RIGER

Community psychology has benefited greatly from adopting theories and methods developed by organizational psychology. Organizational psychologists use multiple perspectives when they analyze organizations: for example, structural theory, a human resources approach, political theories, and cultural analysis (Bolman & Deal, 1984). For community psychologists, then, the organizational perspective contains a wealth of frameworks with which to look at community. Typically, we have adopted these to study advocacy (Riger & Keys, 1987), neighborhood organizations (Wandersman, Florin, Friedmann, & Meier, 1987), and the experience of people who work in social service agencies (Cherniss, 1980; Shinn, Rosario, Morch, & Chestnut, 1984). What we have in common with organizational psychologists (and others) is agreement on a basic paradigmatic assumption (Keys & Frank, 1987a): To understand people, you must understand the settings in which they operate.

Perhaps most important for the field of community psychology, organizational psychologists have developed constructs and measurement techniques that go beyond an individual level of analysis and that can be adapted to community research. For example, Mulvey, Linney, and Rosenberg (1987) use the concept of the distribution of decision-making power within an organization in an examination of residential treatment programs for juvenile offenders. Their description of organizational control is based on Tanenbaum's (1974) notion of the distribution of decision-making power in industry. Gruber and Trickett (1987), in their study of an innovative high school, also use the concept of decision-making power within an organization as a definition of empowerment. Both of these studies demonstrate the usefulness to community research of conceptualizations of the setting that have been developed by organizational psychologists.

Yet the concordance between organizational and community psychology ends when one considers the underlying values and goals of each field. Values that distinguish community psychology from organizational psychology lead us to emphasize the well-being of individuals rather than the organization's efficiency or effectiveness (see Keys & Frank, 1987, and Shinn & Perkins, in press, for excellent overviews of the organizational–community interface). Organizational psychology has as its purpose the identification of ways to improve organizational functioning, typically by looking at middle-level managerial strategies. Critics describe its goal as figuring out how to get more work for less pay out of fewer people (Nord, 1974), whereas supporters argue that organizational psychologists are often the sole defenders of the quality of work life in organizations (Keys, personal communication, 1988). Although interventions that make organizations more effective may incidentally increase job satisfaction or improve working conditions (Shinn & Perkins, in press), that is not their primary purpose.

The values that inform community psychology ought to lead us in a different direction, with a different purpose. We ought to look at those who are on the bottom of the organizational heap—at those who are most affected by organizational practices and policies but who have not effected those policies because they are subordinates in the organization hierarchy. Our purpose ought to be to give voice to their perspective on the organization: To identify how programs and policies affect the choices that are available, and to articulate the strategies that people use to create meaning, given those options. What is critical is that, in studying their lives, we recognize that people are actors who make choices, not simply passive recipients of our interventions, who either accept or fail to see the worth of our programs. How do people with little formal power make their way within organizations? How do they navigate their way among the networks of organizations that structure modern life? What choices are available, and how do they shape those choices? The answers to these questions require that we listen in a different way than usual—indeed, they require that we *listen* above all.

An example of this kind of research comes from work that I have done recently with a team of researchers at Northwestern University concerning people who have left state mental hospitals (Lewis et al., forthcoming). In this case, the organizations involved were the tangled network of social service agencies connected to state mental hospitals. Among other questions, we asked where people went for help when they had problems. The chronically mentally disabled living

I am grateful to Dan Lewis for comments on numerous iterations of the manuscript of this chapter, to Shula Reinharz for introducing me to issues of epistemology in science, and to the editors for helpful suggestions. Revisions of my original paper were stimulated by conference presentations and discussions among participants.

in community settings today suffer from a multiplicity of problems typical of poor, unemployed people: lack of adequate housing, a shortage of jobs, poor health care, and so on. We found that, for many people, especially those who are younger and those who are Black, the family remains the primary source of help. This is true even when people have had multiple hospital admissions and are connected to a social service agency. The only public services used with any frequency were public aid or social security. Thus, from the consumers' point of view of the "organization" of care, social services are much less relevant as supports than family. However, policies are usually aimed at and programs developed for the individual patient. Policies and programs assume that those needing mental health services are autonomous individuals, floating alone through the world. Although this is true of some, in many cases the family may be the unit in crisis. If we shift our perspective slightly and ask what the person's inability to function has done to the family as an organization, we see a different set of needs and possibilities, for example, for support groups for families of the chronically mentally ill such as the Alliance for Mental Illness. The organizational elements under consideration may be the same, but, by shifting the perspective slightly from the program to the person, we can see different patterns and advisable solutions. In understanding what happens when people intersect with policies and programs, too often an organizational approach can take the policy as a given and see if it works or does not work according to its stated goals. What community psychologists using organizational frameworks should do instead is start with people's lives and see how the policy affects what happens to them. Research from this perspective would help reduce the frequency with which we "stumble over our ignorance" of what actually happens to people affected by mental health policies (Shadish, 1984).

Too often, the voices of those subordinate in organizations are not heard in the debate about policies and programs. They are not heard for at least two reasons. First, people who are members of subordinate groups often do not believe that they have the right to speak out. Rodriguez presents an eloquent statement of this in this autobiography, *Hunger of Memory* (1982). Rodriguez, born to a working-class Hispanic family in California, felt that he had no right to a public persona—in his case, to speak out at school—unless and until he became a mainstream American by adopting the English language and rejecting Spanish. Only by becoming Americanized could he speak out, and only in English could his voice be heard by society (see also Sennet & Cobb, 1973).

The second reason why those in subordinate positions are not heard is that those who predominate have the power to define the terms of the discussion and provide explanations for the behavior of people who are lower in a hierarchical relationship (Becker, 1967; Miller, 1986). The superordinate group has more credibility in the public debate, and its explanations are accepted as "truth." Often dominant-group members have preconceived ideas of what should be happening (what we term *hypotheses*), listen only for whether others fit or do not fit those notions, and fail to hear what else is going on. Thus, in the mental health field, we have numerous studies that document the "failure" of deinstitutionalization because mentally disabled people leave the community so often to return to mental hospitals (Kalifon, 1985). What goes unrecognized is the way in which the hospital and allied agencies have become "the community" for people, given the absence of other choices and resources.

IMPLICATIONS FOR ORGANIZATIONAL RESEARCH

If we are to hear the viewpoints of those who are in subordinate positions in organizations, we must go about our research in a different way than business as usual. Our research methods are not well suited to this task. The values of "normal science" emphasize prediction and control for the purpose of dominating nature, and the methods embody separation and distance from that which we are studying. However, to understand another's world from his or her perspective requires empathy, sensitivity to context, acceptance of complexity, and interrelationship rather than domination. Without these qualities, we simply replicate people's everyday experience of subordination within our research; rather than reflecting objectivity, we reflect the status quo (for more extensive discussions of these issues, see Becker, 1967; Bleir, 1984; Keller, 1985; Mischler, 1979; Oakley, 1981; Reinharz, 1979).

How, then, shall we go about doing organizational community research? Guidelines for a new methodology come from feminist scholarship, in particular from a book titled *Women's Ways of Knowing*. (Goldberger, Clinchy, Belenky, & Tarule, 1986). The authors begin the book by raising difficult questions: "What is truth?" "What is authority?" "What counts for me as evidence?" "How do I know what I know?" Although we may frame them in different language, these questions are the central ones with which we grapple as we voice our discontent with research in community psychology. Our answers to these questions define and delimit the research that we do. The authors of *Women's Ways of Knowing* assert that "our basic assumptions about the nature of truth and the origins of knowledge shape the way we see the world and ourselves as participants in it." This is as true for those who do research as for the heterogeneous mix of female students who speak out in interviews in this book.

The authors argue that modes of knowing that are especially common among women differ from those common among men. They identify five epistemological frameworks, linked by the theme of "finding a voice." Typically, scientists use metaphors of vision and sight rather than voice to describe the process of knowledge acquisition. Evelyn Fox Keller (in Belenky et al., 1986) suggests that visual metaphors require passivity on the part of the knower and that distance from the subject is needed to get a proper view. In contrast, hearing and saying implies closeness between subject and object. "Unlike seeing, speaking and listening suggest dialogue and interaction" (Belenky et al., 1986, p. 18). The process of finding a voice is the process of developing the ability and the confidence to participate in the creation of knowledge.

The first of the five epistemological positions identified as typical of women is *silence,* a condition in which women feel neither the right nor the ability to express themselves. The second, *received knowledge,* is a position from which women can accept knowledge from omniscient authorities, but cannot create it on their own. *Subjective knowledge,* the third position, reflects a move from passive to active, from acceptance of external authority to a conception of truth as personal and private, in which one becomes one's own authority. *Procedural knowing,* the fourth position, emphasizes reason and objectivity as strategies for gaining knowledge. It is this position that describes traditional research methods in psychology. The final category is called *constructed knowledge* and has been described as follows:

> The central insight that distinguishes this position is that all knowledge is constructed and the knower is an intimate part of the known. The woman comes to see that the knowledge one acquires depends on the context or frame of reference of the knower who is seeking answers and in the context in which events to be understood have occurred. . . . Empathic seeing and feeling with the other is a central feature of the development of connected knowing. . . . Communion and communication are established with that which one is trying to understand. Women use such images as "conversing with nature," "getting close to ideas," "having rapport with an author" in order to understand, rather than more masculine images such as "pinning an idea down," or "seeing through an argument." (Belenky et al., 1986, p. 216)

The key characteristics of constructed knowledge—that all knowledge is contextual, that knowledge is created by people, and that both objective and subjective strategies are valuable and can be integrated—seem particularly congruent with the values of community psychology. The process of "gaining a voice," of thinking that is informed by feeling rather than devoid of it, of collaborative talk in which new knowledge is developed and ideas emerge, all suggest strategies for community research that extend—indeed, even transform—traditional methodologies.

How, then, do we translate these ideas into research techniques? Suggestions for how to do that come from the description of women at the constructivist level:

> Question posing and problem posing become prominant methods of inquiry. . . . Women tend not to rely as readily or as exclusively on hypothetico-deductive inquiry, which posits an answer (the hypothesis) prior to the data collection, as they do on examining basic assumptions and the conditions in which a problem is cast. For constructivist women, simple questions are as rare as simple answers. Constructivists can take, and often insist upon taking a position outside a particular context or frame of reference and look back on "who" is asking the questions, "why" the question is asked at all, and "how" answers are arrived at (Belenky et al., 1986, p. 139)

Finally, constructivists identify a process of "really talking," rather than didactic talking in which the speaker simply presents ideas to others. "Real talk" is a process of dialogue in which ideas can emerge and be explored, not simply confirmed. Furthermore, the process is collaborative, not hierarchical. "Connected knowing arises out of the experience of relationships; it requires intimacy and equality between self and object, not distance and impersonality; its goal is understanding, not proof" (Belenky et al., 1986, p. 183). "Really talking" suggests to us a method for overcoming silence (see also Reinharz, 1979, on experiential methods). It suggests a process of "dialogue from which knowledge is an unpredictable emergent rather than a controlled outcome" (Westkott, 1979, p. 426). Moreover, it acknowledges that we are linked with those we study in a human relationship and emphasizes the need for an awareness of the ways in which we construct the knowledge that is developed in that context.

The themes that permeate constructivist thought processes are those of connection, mutuality, and reciprocity. These themes are ones that Gilligan (1982) has identified as typifying the way that women (at least in this society at this time) often think about morality. Rather than basing moral decisions on an ethic of rights, they consider responsibilities and care. These themes are particularly evident in the operation of community organizations. At the local level, women are often involved as prime movers of community organizations, and the thrust of their involvement comes from a concern with their families and homes that has been extended to their neighborhoods (Reinharz, 1984). As one organizer put it, "You start by organizing in your house and move to your community" (Chicago Foundation for Women, 1988).

An excellent example of this kind of study of an organization comes from Leavitt and Saegert's (1984) analysis of tenant organizations that formed in buildings that had been abandoned by their owners in Harlem. Moreover, this study exemplifies many of the characteristics of constructivist knowing, of "really talking," and of empathic discourse, in its emphasis on context, on identifying the ways that people shape the resources available to them and the reasons for the choices they make, and on the connection between knowledge and values. Leavitt and Saegert interviewed tenants who were part of a city program that permits people who manage their abandoned building to own it eventually, in a limited equity cooperative arrangement. Many of the leaders of the tenant organizations were female and elderly, and their care of the building extended to care for the sick and elderly tenants. Care for the people in the building is interwoven with care for the physical property:

> . . . communication among the leaders was constant, ways of involving all tenants had been developed, responsibilities were shared maximally and a multidirectional flow of information established. More than this, the ethic of caring for your neighbors extended from relationships among the Board of Directors through the actions of the committee system to look after the sick and elderly through willingness to bear the financial costs of the inability of sick, old people to pay rent increases. (Leavitt & Saegert, 1990, p. 205)

The tenant co-op provided an opportunity for traditional values of women in this community—commitment to community, religious values, and an emphasis on care—to emerge as predominate. These values were extended from the home to encompass the other tenants in a building, in what Leavitt and Saegert call a "community-household model." Neighborhood activism among working-class women often has as its objective the protection of the "welfare of the family-in-the-home-in-the-neighborhood" (Reinharz, 1984). In the community-household model, the welfare of one's own home is assured by protecting the welfare of the building as a whole, as well as the people in it.

One of the critical points that Leavitt and Saegert make is that housing policy is not set up to accommodate this sort of organization. Housing policies assume hierarchical organizational structures where webs exist. "The personal and intensive nature of their approach contrasts with the impersonal, standardized and efficiency-oriented strategies embedded in most housing policies" (Leavitt & Saegert, 1984, p. 38). Existing policy assumes a bureaucratic model of tenant management with values of efficiency and effectiveness, whereas this research suggests a need for policies that are based on nurturance and caring. For example, greater emphasis on maintenance and rehabilitation of buildings rather than on new construction would enable the preservation of existing social relationships. There is little room in current policy for this approach. Furthermore, organizational research that shares the assumptions of the bureaucratic model will not illuminate the presence of supportive webs and how they work.

Both of the studies discussed above are about people in organizations—in one case, the small, personal, nurturing world of a tenants' organization, in the other, the large, often impersonal world of the state mental hospital and associated agencies. What both of these studies have in common is an attempt to enter into the worldview of those whom they are studying, and to see how the organization is experienced from their perspective. These studies take into consideration the context in which people live their lives, the resources they have, and the choices that are available to them. They do not look simply at the effect of a particular program on people, but also consider how that program fits into the totality of people's lives. It is this complexity that we must attempt to capture if we wish to understand the perspective of subordinate groups in organizations.

Doing so will not be easy. We will need to value discovery as well as (and as much as) hypothesis testing; to value exploratory as well as confirmatory research. Yet the biases within the field of psychology make these research strategies deviant—valued by a minority, if at all. Sherif (1987) describes the field of psychology as containing a status hierarchy in which the top rung is occupied by experimentalists, who seek status by aligning their work with the more prestigious physical or natural sciences. The bottom rung is occupied by "applied" researchers. Because this status and value hierarchy prevails in academic departments of psychology, those favoring nonexperimental research strategies, especially on applied topics (as community psychologists are wont to do), will probably be low in status within their departments. Furthermore, because innovations that counter a social system's values and modes of operating are not likely to be adopted (Shadish, 1984), attempts to broaden the range of acceptable methodologies within psychology are likely to be in vain. Indeed, those who resist inclusion of nonexperimental techniques may do so with good reason, because methods such as "constructed knowing" challenge some of the fundamental tenets on which experimentalism is based. Accepting the validity of "constructed knowing" will not simply add more choices to our array of research strategies, but will imply a shift in the value hierarchy within psychology. Given their low status within psychology departments as "applied" researchers, the pressure on many community psychologists is not to innovate but rather to demonstrate acceptability by using research methods that approximate experimental techniques as closely as possible.

Yet psychology departments are not monolithic, and techniques have been accepted in recent years that exemplify some of the characteristics of connected knowing (see e.g., Mitroff, 1983). For example, stakeholder-based evaluation research, a technique that takes consumers' priorities into account in the process of evaluating social programs (Bryk, 1983), can be applied to organizations. This technique attempts to incorporate into the evaluation process questions formulated by the different constituencies that have an interest in the results of an evaluation, especially those who are the least powerful (Mark & Shotland, 1985). In doing so, it implicitly views organizations as political entities, composed of shifting groups with different interests, that compete for scarce resources (Bolman & Deal, 1984). Because stakeholders may differ, the evaluator must decide which group's (or groups') questions will be addressed, bringing the issue of values to the fore. The awareness of the choice process involved reflects an awareness of the way in which knowledge is socially constructed (see Mark & Shotland, 1985).

The limitations of this evaluation strategy may apply to connected knowing as well: Findings may not be generalizable to other settings; the degree of involvement required by the research process may not be practical or desirable from the participants' point of view; and diverse participants may experience a setting in conflicting ways, some of which do not get included (Cook & Shadish, 1986). Descriptive research may limit our ability to make causal inferences. Furthermore, we need to look not only at how individuals experience an organization, but also at the organizational factors that shape and inform individuals' experience (see chapter 11 by Shinn, in this volume, on multiple levels of analysis). Finally, simply giving voice to the experience of the least powerful in organizations may not lead to change (Mark & Shotland, 1985).

Although these difficulties may place limits on the constructivist approach, transformation of research methods to include this way of knowing would bring us closer to our goal of assessing the impact of organizations on people's lives rather than simply viewing people as organizational components. Each of the major theoretical perspectives in organizational psychology examines a different set of issues. Structural theory directs us to examine the way in which jobs are organized and activity is integrated; a human relations approach focuses on individual needs, skills, and attitudes toward one's job; a political approach examines the shifting set of coalitions and alliances that make up organizational life; and the symbolic approach examines organizations as a stage upon which dramas are enacted that reflect human needs and concerns (Bolman & Deal, 1984). Within each of these frameworks, the use of constructivist research methods will let us examine the impact of the organization on its members in a manner that permits consideration of the complexity of human experience. It will facilitate elucidation of the impact of the organization on those at the bottom of the organization's hierarchy, particularly those who are the recipients of its services. As Seidman (1983) states, in a discussion of social problem solving, "[r]ecipients, who are presumed to benefit in the short or long run, can no longer be excluded or incorporated in only token fashion if the process is to be truly meaningful and beneficial to them. They may have dramatically different conceptualizations" (p. 66). Constructivist knowing is an approach to research that will enable recipients' conceptualizations of the organization to become part of the discussion. It is a way for community psychologists to apply organizational frames to the aspects of organizational processes that we value knowing about.

In a planning discussion for the conference on which this book is based, the felicitous phrase "criteria for adventuresome research" became a touchstone of what we hoped to accomplish. The lack of adventuresome research in community psychology is deplored every few years when some of our colleagues muster the energy to review all of the articles published in one of our journals (Loo, Fong, & Iwamasa, 1988; Lounsbury, Leader, Meares, & Cook, 1980; McClure et al. 1980; Novaco & Monahan, 1980). It is not simply that we lack the imagination to translate our values and beliefs into research questions. Rather, our adherence to traditional scientific methods limits what we can study, and what we hear.

I do not advocate the elimination of discipline and conscientiousness in our research; nor am I suggesting that we reject quantitative methods (as the example of stakeholder analysis above demonstrates). Rather, let us retain the best qualities of current research methods and expand them, transforming them in the process. Traditional research methods, as reflective of mainstream American culture, emphasize objectivity, efficiency, separateness, and distance. Yet objectivity need not be confounded with domination or hierarchical relations with those whom we study (Keller, 1985). Let us consider as well connection and empathy as modes of knowing and embrace them in our criteria and in our work. We would do well to make room for "constructed knowing" in our adventuresome research.

CHAPTER 6

RESEARCH METHODS AND THE EMPOWERMENT SOCIAL AGENDA

JULIAN RAPPAPORT

> As for the scientists who enter the arena of social action . . . they would do well to be guided by the values they attach to the facts of living. . . . This will present scientists with a type of problem (and transform their concepts of solution) for which their scientific models are inappropriate and may even be interfering. They will find themselves dealing in persuasion, not only in facts; the problems will change before and within them; they will not be concerned with replicability because that will be impossible; there will be no final solutions, only a constantly upsetting imbalance between values and action; the internal conflict will not be in the form of "Do I have the right answer?" but rather "Am I being consistent with what I believe?"; satisfaction will come not from colleagues' consensus that their procedures, facts, and conclusions are independent of their feelings and values, but from their own convictions that they tried to be true to their values; they will fight to win not in order to establish the superiority of their procedures or the validity of their scientific facts, concepts and theories, but because they want to live with themselves and others in certain ways. (Sarason, 1978, p. 379)

In two previous publications (Rappaport, 1981, 1987) I have made the case for adoption of an empowerment agenda as the phenomenon of interest for theory development, as the goal of social and community intervention, and as an organizing force for maintaining community psychology as a social movement. Here I intend to raise some research implications for those who do hold an empowerment social agenda and who, in Sarason's words quoted above, "want to live with themselves and others in certain ways" consistent with their values.

A BRIEF STATEMENT OF THE EMPOWERMENT AGENDA

To be committed to an empowerment social agenda and to be consistent with that agenda in one's approach to social science theory, research, and action is to be committed to identifying, facilitating, or creating contexts in which heretofore silent and isolated people, those who are "outsiders" in various settings, organizations, and communities, gain understanding, voice, and influence over decisions that affect their lives.[1] Empowerment is by definition concerned with many who are excluded by the majority society on the basis of their demographic characteristics or of their physical or emotional difficulties, experienced either in the past or the present. Such people are often allotted a low *ascribed* status, and are afforded little opportunity to attain *achieved* status (Sarbin, 1970). Thus, for those who are society's outsiders, the issues of empowerment will be different than for other more advantaged groups. Adoption of an empowerment agenda should make researchers sensitive to such matters. The term loses its meaning if it is applied without such concerns. (A more elaborated statement of the empowerment agenda appears elsewhere; Rappaport, 1981, 1984, 1985, & 1987.)[2]

The empowerment agenda will have a number of implications for research methodology. Although the implications are methodological in nature, they do not specify particular research designs, measures, or data-analysis techniques. They do concern themselves with how to conduct research (rather than what to research) and could be applied to most content areas. They become figure rather than ground for those who hold to an empowerment social agenda, regardless of what one is studying. Those who hold empowerment social values, regardless of the particular content of the research, will confront a variety of contradictions between the usual ways of conducting research and those that are implied by their values.

Preparation of this chapter benefited from Research Grant MH37390 from the National Institute of Mental Health and from collaboration with many members of GROW, Inc., an international mutual-help organization for people with a history of mental illness. My appreciation is extended to Brad Heil, Douglas Luke, Mellen Kennedy, Joyce Pfenning, Richard Ziegler, and, especially, Marc Zimmerman for comments on an earlier version.

[1]There is probably too much jargon in this agenda statement. I am often asked what do I really mean by *empowerment?* I admit to a certain lack of precision in the term. For example, one might be asked to define things like *context, influence,* and *decisions.* And it would be helpful to specify just what is meant by a phrase such as *affect their lives.* Nevertheless, despite the difficulty of specification I have discovered that it is not very difficult for the people who are the target of our research or our interventions to understand what it means. Empowerment has also been written about by political scientists, journalists, and poets (e.g., Boyte & Reissman, 1986; Neruda, 1987).

[2]Of course, this does not mean that outsiders should be the only people studied. One may learn quite a bit by studying those who are empowered "insiders" and by studying settings that are empowering (Maton, 1989; Maton & Rappaport, 1984) as well as people who have become empowered (Kieffer, 1984). There are also certain uses that, although not totally congruent with the intention to retain the term *empowerment* for issues concerned with outsiders, do not distort its meaning and from which we probably can learn a great deal—for example, empowering teachers or parents in the school context (see Gruber & Trickett, 1987).

CONFRONTING CONTRADICTIONS

Those who hold scientific power—government funding agencies, foundations, journal editors—tend to hold a uniform view of what constitutes acceptable scientific method, leading some philosophers of science (e.g., Feyerabend, 1978) to suggest that the defense of freedom is now less a question of separation of church and state than a problem of how to separate science from state. In other words, methods tend to be a priori considered better or worse according to a standard that cuts across the content studied, the intention of the research, or the social values of the researcher. That the method of study can change our understanding of the content is considered an annoying but not a central issue. That it can actually change the content itself (not merely our understanding of it) is rarely considered. However, doing research does change the thing studied, especially if what is studied is people. How we conduct the research, what we conceptualize and communicate to and about the people of concern, directly and indirectly changes more than what we find out—it also actually changes the people we study.[3]

Because research changes those who participate in it, those who hold empowerment social values may find that they need to engage in certain methodological practices that contradict those currently popular in mainstream psychology. Unfortunately, many otherwise acceptable scientific practices (e.g., treating the people of concern as "subjects") are often inconsistent with an empowerment social agenda, while a variety of practices (e.g., genuine collaboration with research participants) that are consistent with empowerment intentions are by their very nature questionable under currently popular scientific canons.

Intelligent discussions of the role of scientists and of their responsibility to be problem-oriented experimenters who evaluate and disseminate innovations in socially responsible ways have been presented (e.g., Fairweather & Davidson, 1986), but the relationship between values and method per se (how one studies as a function of what one values) is not, with the exception of a feminist critique (e.g., Belenky, Clinchy, Goldberger, & Tarule, 1986; Gilligan, 1982), typically discussed. Even when admitting that there is no value-free science, one usually expresses a faith in *the* scientific method, which is applicable regardless of the content to which it is applied. An empowerment social agenda asks that the means of acquiring data do not contradict the aims of empowerment, regardless of the content of the research.

The values of empowerment suggest that our work should benefit society's outsiders. The work should be done in the context of the people of concern. It

---

[3]That the social science community has adopted certain traditions and ethical principles vis-à-vis deception, for example, attests to the fact that most of us believe that there is an impact of how we do research on the human beings whom we study. Especially in contexts other than university courses and laboratories, we may require certain other safeguards for ethics beyond what is now called *informed consent*. A discussion of these ethical issues is beyond the scope of the present chapter, although they will ultimately influence many of the issues raised here (cf. O'Neill, 1989).

should be collaborative and oriented toward strengths rather than deficits. It should give voice to the people of concern, allow for paradoxical and qualitative understanding, and seek descriptive authenticity. The remainder of this chapter explores such issues. The intention is to increase the likelihood that our research methodology will be consistent with our social values.

RESEARCH DESIGN SHOULD CONSIDER WHO BENEFITS FROM THE RESEARCH

The first question that must be taken seriously by those who hold an empowerment ideology is, For whose benefit is this research conducted? This question is not answered by the standard rationalization that such matters are not of concern to scientists. For those who hold empowerment values, how it is answered is as much a part of methodology as the selection of measures and data-analytic procedures. Like all methodological issues the question calls for an answer that requires forethought and decision on the part of the researcher. The answer to the question of who the research will be designed to benefit is a matter of choice, and, like all methodological choices, it tells us something about the researcher's priorities.

There is rarely any question that the scientist's research is designed to benefit the scientist or the scientist's career. There is little point in being embarrassed about that. We usually say it also benefits others, but it is often unclear how or whom, except in some abstract sense of potential future benefit to unspecified others from knowledge gained. This lack of clarity is a serious problem for those who care to raise it. One is at risk of sounding anti-intellectual if one asks, "Who benefits from this research?" and expects a serious answer rather than a rationalization about long-term contributions to knowledge. Nevertheless, much knowledge obtained from social science research is noncumulative and quickly forgotten, benefiting only the people who do research for a living. Of course, we cannot always know ahead of time which research will pay off with a cumulative contribution, so we cannot say before the fact which research is worth doing. To do so would be anti-intellectual, bad science, and bad politics. Often, however, we can know about the immediate benefit or harm to the people whom we study. It is quite possible to conduct research that is equally likely (or unlikely) to have long-term benefits for the accumulation of knowledge as well as obvious immediate benefit for the people of concern. In other words, research from an empowerment ideology suggests that we consider both the long-term abstract potential benefit to knowledge and the likelihood that the research will be consistent with empowerment of the people of concern. There is no reason why these considerations cannot both be the aims of our research. An empowerment ideology implies that we must justify our research both in terms of its potential as a contribution to knowledge and in terms of its empowering impact on the people who participate in it.

RESEARCH SHOULD BE CONDUCTED IN THE CONTEXT OF THE PEOPLE OF CONCERN

To be committed to empowerment is to be an action-researcher—one who identifies, facilitates, creates. That is what action-researchers do. To say that we do this with respect to contexts is to make a theoretical, a methodological, and an action statement. Some things are difficult to study or influence out of context. For example, if one wants to know about community life, it is probably helpful to see people in their community settings. This does not mean one can never learn from talking to people away from their communities, or from observing how they behave in research settings. But if one wants to know about behavior in a community, studying persons out of their own context imposes certain limitations, despite the advantage of convenience and control that it affords the researcher. Something is gained, and something is lost. The choice matters, and it suggests priorities.

Community psychologists began with the assumption that professional services in hospitals, clinics, and consulting room settings are of limited value to many clients of concern, despite the advantage of convenience and prestige to the professional caregiver. Oddly, we have been slower to recognize the same constraints on research setting and on methods. An empowerment priority leads one to work with people in their own context because we assume that doing so is the best science as well as the best practice. This assumption is exactly the opposite of the assumption that we should study and help people in our consulting rooms and laboratories because that is where we do the best helping and the best science. In and of itself, neither of these assumptions is correct. The empowerment agenda, for both a sound research reason (these are the contexts that are most interesting to us and those to which we hope our work will apply) and for a sound service reason (people are more likely to benefit from programs delivered in the context of their everyday life), starts with the assumption that working with people in their own context is the best option. One ought to have a very good reason, other than convenience, for taking people out of context.

COLLABORATIVE RESEARCH BEGINS BEFORE THE BEGINNING

Currently acceptable dominant research methods encourage researchers to treat the person studied as a "subject" and to remain "objective" unless there is some reason why to do so is impossible. Empowerment ideology suggests the opposite: We should encourage the researcher to collaborate with research participants unless there is some good reason not to do so. From the empowerment perspective, it is wrong to assume that distancing oneself from research participants is always the best way to know anything useful. If the research method is itself disempowering (e.g., by disregarding the constructed reality of a participant), the process of doing the research may be more likely to contribute to a degrading rather than to an empowering outcome, particularly if the person studied has a stake in the research findings. In short, for the empowerment researcher collaboration must be part of the research design—it begins "before the beginning" (Sarason, 1972).

Even research within the constraints of our dominant methodology can be consistent with an empowering intention if the researcher is sensitive to such issues. For example, Wood, Taylor, and Lichtman (1985), in a study of women with breast cancer, published in the mainstream *Journal of Personality and Social Psychology,* were interested in testing certain theoretical questions with respect to social comparison processes. As the research proceeded, they used an interview technique that enabled them to communicate with the women and to obtain more than the limited information provided by their objective rating scales. Recording the interviews enabled the researchers later to code responses so as to achieve a broader understanding of the constructs that they sought to grasp. In addition to looking for positive ways in which these women were active copers, they avoided an exclusive focus on seeing them as victims of hardships. Such a methodology has a higher likelihood than a rigidly structured survey or questionnaire of enabling the researcher to interact with the participant in ways that change them both. In this case, the researchers gave to the participants a sense of their ability to influence not only themselves but also the researchers. It should be noted that these researchers never mention the word *empowerment* in their report. Empowerment need not be the explicit topic of all research for us to expect, as a matter of methodology (just as we consider issues of research design and data analysis to apply to all research), that the procedures themselves should be empowering rather than disempowering, should focus the individuals who are studied on more than their weaknesses, and should enable the participants to have a positive sense of influence on the researcher.

This example is suggested as a minimum standard. For those who want to study and to enhance empowerment per se, more is needed. A collaborative relationship with the people of interest begins at the conception of the research, so as to give voice to participants' definitions of reality (Rappaport et al., 1985; Cf. Reinharz, 1988). An empowerment agenda suggests that the research methodology should be both congruent with the values and goals of the research and collaborative, in the sense that participants should have an opportunity to influence the conception, the measures, and the procedures even before the data are collected.

If we are willing to collaborate with the targets of our work—be they those people whom we study, those to whom we try to be helpful, or both—the meaning of empowerment becomes quite clear. We know and they know when what we are doing is empowering to them and when it is not. To take advantage of this knowledge requires listening to the people with whom we are working and studying. It means respecting their "experiential knowledge" (Borkman, 1990). It means adopting their perspective as well as our own. Both parties know when understanding or a sense of personal agency has taken place. (We may need to worry about how to define and measure such understanding for research purposes, but that is a different problem.)

To say that collaboration is important is to say something about the relationship between the action-researcher and the persons of concern. That is, when people genuinely collaborate, they engage in a mutual-influence process that involves each listening to the other, processing communications in good faith, and reevaluating their own views in light of the views of the other. This process requires mutual respect and a willingness to be shaped as well as to be a shaper. Such a mutual-influence relationship is rare between helper and helpee, and even rarer between researcher and subject (as is implied by the terms that we give to those with whom we work). A *client,* a *patient,* or a *subject* is one who is expected to change, get better, or perform for the researcher who manipulates things. At first blush, one might assume that professionals and researchers are not expected to change as a function of their interactions with such people. But isn't research about learning new things? And, if we do learn, shouldn't we change too? Perhaps research and collaboration are more compatible than we have been led to believe.

We can learn from collaboration (which requires us to regard the other as a partner), and we can learn from objectifying (regarding the subject as an object). In either case, we should expect to be changed persons if we have had a successful research experience. Collaboration can facilitate the learning process in ways that are different from those resulting from objectification. Something is gained and something is lost in either approach. However, it is not necessary to objectify in order to learn something. So-called clinical methods, those that force us to pay attention to the experiential knowledge of people that we study, to our own intuitions, and to our relationship with each other, can be applied to social and organizational research (e.g., Berg & Smith, 1988) as well as to research concerned with individuals.

EMPOWERING RESEARCH IS BASED ON A STRENGTHS PERSPECTIVE THAT GIVES VOICE TO THE PEOPLE OF CONCERN

Assessment always distorts by presenting a limited perspective. All research distorts, but some methods do so more than others; and no two methods distort in exactly the same way. We acknowledge this distortion when we speak about the need for a "critical multiplism methodology" (Shadish, 1986a). However, we rarely concern ourselves with it as a matter of impact on the people that we study. Different distortions not only give us different data, they also empower different actors. If we have rarely asked the question of whom the content of this research empowers, we have even more rarely asked the following important questions: Who does this method of research empower? What voice does it amplify? Whose point of view does it champion?

From an empowerment perspective, the contexts that we identify to study, facilitate, or create indicate a choice as to whose voice we consider to be important. As suggested above, to choose empowerment is to choose an option in favor of the poor, the powerless, and the dispossessed. By design, one will often be on the side of inmates, mental patients, ethnic and racial minorities, economically poor people, the physically limited, and, in many cases, women. Research guided by an empowerment agenda will therefore use a methodology consistent with such goals. The context of the research will be the context of the people of concern, and the assessment methodology that is used will frame the issues and see the world from their viewpoint. It is their voice that we wish to amplify (Reinharz, 1988).

As we do so, we must assume a strengths perspective. That is, rather than concerning ourselves with deficits or finding out what is wrong with people and trying to fix matters, we must look for abilities and skills and seek to identify, facilitate, or create contexts in which each person's capacities may become figure rather than ground. In a world defined by single standards imposed by others, those of us concerned with empowerment seek greater diversity and more varied rules for access to material, social, and psychological resources. We assume that every person has certain strengths.

By definition we are always looking for the obvious or hidden strengths of the people that we study so that both they and we can learn from them. The metacommunication to the people with whom we work is, "You are a competent person." Open to research are such questions as: How do we identify, facilitate, and create contexts that empower by facilitating the use of the strengths people already possess? How do settings that seem to empower people operate? What are the mechanisms, at various levels of analysis, that lead to the empowerment of people?

The methodological point of a strengths perspective speaks to both theory and assessment. It places demands on both what is measured and how it is measured. To adopt a strengths perspective forces us to look for what is competent and important in each person. It means we must get to know something about the people we study in their own context before we attempt to do research. For example, people who are economically poor will have a variety of skills and ideas that they can use to attain resources. Those who are identified as mental patients will have many abilities to which their psychiatric status will be irrelevant. The communities and settings in which people live will have many assets and resources that can be mobilized once identified. To work within an empowering ideology requires us to identify (for ourselves, for others, and for the people with whom we work) the abilities they possess that may not be obvious, even to themselves. That is the point of our research. It is always easier to see what is wrong and what people lack. Empowering research attempts to identify what is right with people and what resources are already available, so as to encourage their use and expansion under the control of the people of concern.

Research that asserts a strengths perspective and that seeks to give voice to the people of concern may benefit from data-collection and analysis approaches that emphasize description, multiple perspectives, and authentication of those voices that are often ignored. Two such methods are suggested below.

Paradoxical Criteria for Program Evaluation May Give Voice to the People of Concern

This suggestion is taken from Cameron (1986), an organizational psychologist writing about why organizational effectiveness is inherently paradoxical. He argues that the most effective organizations are those characterized by paradoxes—"contradictory, mutually exclusive elements that are present and operate equally at the same time" (p. 545). He asserts that because different constituencies hold sometimes opposite preferences and expectations, the most effective organizations often perform in contradictory ways. This is, of course, a point of view that is philosophically consistent with much of the previous writing on empowerment, including the importance of divergent reasoning, the eschewing of single standards of competence and of single solutions to social problems (see Rappaport, 1977, 1981, for an extended discussion of this point of view). It is also consistent with a research methodology that calls for at least two differing perspectives in the same study (Seidman, 1978; Zane & Sue, 1986).

One of the implications for research to which Cameron points is that, in organizations, the criteria of effectiveness may be independent of the criteria of ineffectiveness, just as in studies of health, high scores on indicators of wellness may indicate health, but low scores do not necessarily indicate illness. Applying this sort of thinking allows us to see that the criteria for positive outcomes from any social program may be different for those who are the gatekeepers and authorities than for those who are the outsiders. Poor performance on one set of criteria does not necessarily imply poor performance on the other. For example, evaluating preschool programs only in terms of IQ scores may lead to different conclusions than evaluating such programs in terms of the child-care needs of the parents. In research, both perspectives need to be conceptualized, measured, and represented in analysis as well as in policy recommendations.

Statistical procedures may obscure the existence of paradoxical criteria, and so fail to give voice to the people of concern. Some years ago, Bergin (1966) suggested that psychotherapy research that is based on group mean comparisons between treatment and control groups may mask the reality that on a given measure, some people will improve, others get worse, and others remain stable. He pointed out that it is quite possible that half of those in a treatment group will improve and the other half get worse, while the comparison group remains stable. Comparing group means can hide the individual variability and, thus, suggest no change in the treatment group when there is actually a great deal of change—for better or for worse. Cameron (1986) notes that "taking averages and finding midpoints may mask the presence of paradox, as might the reliance on linear trends in regression equations" (p. 551). He suggests that outliers and contradictions should not be neglected and that, as Tukey (1977) suggested, data should be explored in nonstatistical ways. One may also apply certain statistical techniques, for example, cluster analysis, to describe different groups of people or settings (cf. Luke, 1988; Salem, 1988) within a particular context (see chapter 13a, by Rapkin & Mulvey, in this volume).

Naturalistic qualitative analysis (discussed below) is also consistent with this research approach and may be a path toward combining qualitative and quantitative methodologies (e.g., Miles & Huberman, 1984). From an empowerment perspective, a methodology that not only recognizes diversity and multiple perspectives, but also looks for them, is highly desirable.

Naturalistic Research May Help Give Voice to the People of Concern

Lincoln and Guba, qualitative researchers concerned with educational evaluation, provide a methodological framework consistent with the empowerment social agenda. They summarize (1986) a viewpoint developed in the context of naturalistic evaluation in educational settings. Their axioms for "naturalistic and responsive evaluations" include the following assumptions: There are multiple and constructed realities; human behavior is time- and context-bound, to the extent that enduring context-free generalization is impossible; application of findings from one setting to another requires a detailed comparison only possible when the setting (context) is "thickly described"; causality is multifactored and multidirectional; the researcher cannot be objective; the relationship between the researcher and the persons of concern is one of "respectful negotiation, joint control, and reciprocal learning" (Lincoln & Guba, 1986, p. 76). Clearly, this viewpoint is consistent with the philosophical assumptions of the empowerment agenda described here and elsewhere (Rappaport, 1981, 1987; Seidman, 1978; Seidman & Rappaport, 1986).

Lincoln and Guba (1986) describe two approaches to the development of criteria for naturalistic research. One, referred to as *trustworthiness,* is intended to parallel the dominant research approach, which calls for internal and external validity, reliability, and objectivity. They propose substitute criteria, which they call *credibility, transferability, dependability,* and *confirmability.* Techniques for meeting these criteria include prolonged engagement, persistent observation, triangulation of sources and methods, negative case analysis, member checks, thick (very detailed) description to enable others to compare the setting with their own, and an external audit. These parallel criteria are summarized according to their trustworthiness function and placed in comparison to the dominant paradigm in Table 1 (see also Lincoln & Guba, 1985, for more detail).

Perhaps more important, these authors also propose a "unique criterion of authenticity" that is largely ignored by the dominant paradigm but is intrinsic to the sort of philosophical assumptions described in the first paragraph of this section, which I believe to be consistent with an empowerment agenda. Their

Table 1

PARALLEL CRITERIA FOR TRUSTWORTHINESS IN NATURALISTIC
RESEARCH APPLICABLE TO AN EMPOWERMENT AGENDA

Basic questions	Dominant paradigm criteria for rigor	To obviate the problem of:	With the technique of:	Parallel naturalistic criteria for trustworthiness
Truth value	**Internal validity**	Confounding	Control or randomization	**Credibility** Prolonged engagement and observation, triangulation of sources and methods; negative case analysis and member checks
Applicability	**External validity**	Atypicality	Representative sampling	**Transferability** Thick (detailed) description to permit others to determine similarity to new contexts
Consistency	**Reliability**	Instability	Replication	**Dependability** External audit of the process by a competent disinterested party
Neutrality	**Objectivity**	Bias	Insulation	**Confirmability** External audit of the product

Note. This table is a summary, constructed with the assistance of Mellen Kennedy from the work of Lincoln and Guba (1986). Although the table was drawn for this chapter, the ideas are those of Lincoln and Guba and are adapted here with the authors' permission.

criteria include what they term *fairness, ontological authentication, educational authentication, catalytic authentication,* and *tactical authenticity* (Table 2). What they suggest is not a set of techniques, but what they hope will be a useful heuristic for consideration. These criteria are highly important to the empowerment researcher.

As to fairness, they are concerned that, in any evaluation, the various values, belief systems, and constructions of all stakeholders must be represented. With respect to program evaluation recommendations, negotiation must be openly carried out by skilled, equally powerful actors who represent the various points of view. Information must be available to all parties of concern, on the basis of informed consent and continuous involvement and feedback to the people of concern. Thus, collaboration, as we have defined it here, is essential for fairness.

Table 2

UNIQUE CRITERIA OF AUTHENTICITY FOR NATURALISTIC RESEARCH
CONSISTENT WITH AN EMPOWERMENT AGENDA

Criterion	Definition
Fairness	Representation of all stakeholder's constructions of reality; open negotiations among equally powerful actors; all information available to all stakeholders; informed involvement; continuous feedback and collaboration
Ontological authentication	Raised consciousness of all parties, including the researcher, as to complexities of social, political, and cultural factors
Educational authentication	Enhanced understanding of the realities of others; particular concern with the education of gatekeepers
Catalytic authentication	Inquiry, understanding, and action are part of a collaborative whole that gives "voice to the speechless"
Tactual authenticity	Evaluation includes the question "To whom is this research empowering?"; people of concern are collaborators in the use of information acquired, not subjects to whom it is applied

Note. This table is a summary, constructed with the assistance of Mellen Kennedy from the work of Lincoln and Guba (1986). Although the table was drawn for this chapter, the ideas are those of Lincoln and Guba and are adapted here with the authors' permission.

By *ontological authentication,* Lincoln and Guba mean raising the consciousness of all parties, including the researcher, as to the complexity of social, cultural, and political factors that have, in this context. shaped the views of the various actors. *Educational authentication* means enabling people to understand the constructed realities of other actors in the setting. For example, those in gatekeeping positions of power and control ought to come to understand the ideas and experiences of others better. The notion of giving voice to the heretofore disempowered is consistent with this objective.

Catalytic authentication refers to the requirement that inquiry and understanding lead to action. In their words:

> The naturalistic posture that involves all stakeholders from the start, that honors their inputs, that provides them with decisionmaking power in guiding the evaluation, that attempts to empower the powerless and give voice to the speechless, and that results in a collaborative effort hold[s] more promise (than calls for theory into action and federal programs for dissemination of research) for eliminating such hoary distinctions as basic versus applied and theory versus practice (Lincoln & Guba, 1986, p. 82).

Finally, *tactical authenticity* is a concern with the real outcomes of the research process. "Chief among these is the matter of whether the evaluation is empowering or impoverishing, and to whom" (Lincoln & Guba, 1986, p. 82).

Consistent with my argument here, Lincoln and Guba suggest that respondents ought not to be treated as subjects to be manipulated, treated, or deceived in the interest of some "good." Tactical authenticity requires collaboration in all things.

Such criteria, although emphasizing naturalistic qualitative analysis, do not exclude quantitative methods. Rather, they add certain positive elements to the construction, administration, and conduct of the research process. They encourage certain additional methods before, during, and after the formal research process. They involve the people of concern in the planning, the construction of measures, and the carrying out of the project in more ways that enhance its implementation. They assure representation of the constructed reality of the people of concern in the initial conception, analysis, and drawing of conclusions, as well as in the use to which the information is put.

CONCLUSION

This chapter has been concerned with some orienting assumptions and implications for research practices that are consistent with an empowerment agenda. Much of the concern has been with the "how" of doing research rather than with the content. I have assumed that, when an empowerment agenda is adopted by the researcher, the salient issue becomes how, as Sarason suggests in the quote at the beginning of this chapter, to live with ourselves and others in certain ways consistent with such an agenda. Although the implications presented are an incomplete listing and have not dealt with the considerable barriers to doing such research, they offer a number of methodological issues for consideration before the beginning of any research project. The time to consider these methodological issues is when the research design, measures, data collection, and analysis procedures are being planned: In what context will the research be conducted? Who will benefit? Whose voices will be heard? How will the work accomplish authenticity? How can the people of concern be genuine collaborators? How can the researchers find the strengths in people and in communities? How can the researchers develop paradoxical criteria for outcomes representing different constituencies? How can the researchers use alternative statistical methods as well as qualitative ones? For those who hold an empowerment social agenda, such questions can lead to an exciting adventure in new ways of doing research.

CHAPTER 7

SOME EMERGING STANDARDS FOR COMMUNITY RESEARCH AND ACTION:
AID FROM A BEHAVIORAL PERSPECTIVE

STEPHEN B. FAWCETT

In the late 1960s I worked as a VISTA Volunteer and community organizer on Kansas City's west side. High on ideals and low on competence, I was awed by the complexity of the public housing project in which I lived and deeply moved by the pain and joy of the people whose lives I came to know. My personal quest to understand this experience—and to have an impact on the conditions that produced the obvious problems in living—led me to two quite divergent books: *Reveille for Radicals* (1969), by community organizer Saul Alinsky, and *Science and Human Behavior* (1953), by behavioral psychologist B. F. Skinner. Reading Alinsky, I was uplifted by the values of social justice and inspired by the small wins these organizing efforts produced. Reading Skinner, I was drawn to the prospects for a natural science of community action that could more reliably contribute to the social good. My marginal status as an outsider in that Kansas City community and these early attempts at synthesis foreshadowed the current challenge of integrating alternate models of community psychology into a set of standards for community research and action.

Standards are valued when they help us see common ground, enable us to detect whether something measures up, and inspire us to reach beyond our present grasp. The literal meaning of *standard,* a standing place, should serve as a caution, however, against being governed by inflexible rules that limit diversity, fail to detect alternatives, and are otherwise unresponsive to changing goals and contexts. Functional standards for community research and action should outline a common vision, help us select more valued activity and products, and encourage us to aspire to higher levels of excellence and attainment.

A central question in outlining such standards is how community psychology can be both a field of study *about* communities and a field *for* and *with* those communities that we study. Community psychology, like many academic disciplines, places a premium on conceptual and methodological sophistication, devaluing action components that can contribute to improvement and inform theory. We must match our rhetoric about prevention and empowerment with actions that empower people and that prevent the problems in living that we examine. Our challenge is to discover standards that optimize both rigor and relevance in the pursuit of understanding and action.

The purpose of this chapter, then, is to outline some issues in and standards for conducting both research and action with communities. These dimensions constitute an attempted synthesis of the insights of alternate models in traditional community psychology and the behavior-analytic paradigm of community research. Emerging standards for guiding community research and action efforts are outlined, and their implications for the field are noted.

INTEGRATING VARIOUS TRADITIONAL AND BEHAVIOR-ANALYTIC MODELS

We should have no illusions about the ease of producing a synthesis of traditional and behavior-analytic models in community psychology. Ecological, organizational, developmental, and behavior-analytic models have differing world views. Traditional models in community psychology draw attention to the complexity of relations within and between social contexts and seem to suggest that many social problems are intractable (Bogat & Jason, in press). By contrast, the behavior-analytic paradigm focuses (seemingly exclusively) on the objective features of the proximal environment and holds that social problems can be analyzed and solved, although practitioners to acknowledge potential limitations.

The behavior-analytic paradigm views the conditions that people label as social problems as a function of an interaction between the behavior of people (in the territories, organizations, and subcultures that define the community of interest) and the physical and social environmental events (of the proximate and broader context). It would be assumed under this paradigm that welfare dependence and the related behavior of job seeking, for instance, are affected by a

I am grateful to the current and former research collaborators from whom I have learned about community research and action, including the following who commented on this chapter: Fabricio Balcazar, Kathy Blanchard, Melody Embree, Mike Johnson, Mark Mathews, Adrienne Paine, Kay Fletcher Schriner, Tom Seekins, John F. Smith, Yolanda Suarez, and Glen White. I especially want to thank Lenny Jason for his significant contribution to this chapter through an extended dialogue on these issues. In addition, I thank Bill Berkowitz, Brenna Bry, David Chavis, Susan Elkins, David Glenwick, Ken Maton, Bob Newbrough, Rick Price, Tom Welsh, and Mont Wolf for their very helpful reactions to a draft of this chapter.

variety of events antecedent to looking for work, such as information about job openings, and of events consequent to job seeking, including the costs and benefits of working. These include broader structural variables (such as welfare regulations that function as disincentives to working by reducing benefits for health insurance and child care) and such proximate variables as knowledge of job opportunities and participation in social networks that link applicants with people who are able to provide decent jobs. Social interventions derived from that paradigm assume that what can occur depends on the physical structure of the environment, and that what will occur depends on behavior–environment relationships in the current context (see Morris, 1988, for a discussion of the fundamentally contextual nature of behavior analysis).

The behavior-analytic paradigm uses experimental designs to examine the effects of social interventions composed of modifiable variables (such as work incentives, job skills programs) on the behaviors (such as job seeking) and outcomes (such as employment and reduced welfare dependency) valued by client audiences.

I could recite a litany of possible limitations of the behavior-analytic paradigm. However, my colleagues and I have done this elsewhere (e.g., Fawcett, Mathews, & Fletcher, 1980), and each community psychologist may have his or her own cherished list. Our collective list of potential limitations might note interventions that may disrupt beneficial aspects of the context, procedural specifications that may limit flexibility, process and outcome goals that may violate norms of cultural relativity and respect for diversity, and a small-wins orientation that may draw attention away from other needed changes in the larger system that affect behavior and related community conditions.

I could also spell out an apologia for the behavior-analytic paradigm, which might take note of the value of focusing on real behavior of actual members of the community of interest (not analog responses of analog subjects), reliable measurement systems, preference for experimental designs that provide formative evaluations that can be used to improve interventions, effective and replicable social interventions, and attention to environmental features upon which action can be taken. The issue is not whether the list of limitations or of strengths is longer, but rather how the valued contributions of the behavior-analytic paradigm can be forged with other models to produce a stronger paradigm (and a related set of standards) for community research and action.

SOME KEY CONCEPTS IN COMMUNITY RESEARCH AND ACTION

A number of important concepts in the practice of community research and action are suggested by a synthesis of traditional and behavior-analytic models. This section addresses several of them: the question of who the client is, the idea of collaboration, the idea of problem, questions about what levels at which to study, the idea of small wins, values of researchers, and the broader context of research and action.

The basic question—Who is the client?—invites consideration of the legitimacy of the endeavor's constituents. Those permitted to influence the goals for research and action through funding or other relationships constitute our (often implicit) choices of clients. Targets of research—those whose behavior would be understood or changed—should not be confused with clients, whose ends may be furthered by studies. The choice of clients—whether homeless people living on an urban street or the proprietors and residents of nearby stores and homes— provides insight into researchers' values and the prevailing assumptions about which community conditions are truly in the public interest and how societal benefits should be distributed.

The *idea of collaboration,* a major tradition of community psychology, calls for researchers to involve clients as partners in the consultation process (e.g., Kelly, 1986a). It leads researchers to avoid "colonial" relationships with research targets by sharing information and resources and by ensuring that an equitable distribution of benefits results from the research (Chavis, Stuckey, & Wandersman, 1983).

A central issue in collaborative relationships is framed in the question, What goals are valued by the client? This question is made complicated by the recognition that there is no such thing as *the* poor, *the* disabled, or *the* tribe, from whom what is valued by the community of interest can be reliably discerned. We have addressed this problem by using a "concerns report" process that combines quantitative and qualitative methods so as to involve groups of disadvantaged people in setting issue agendas and identifying acceptable alternatives for action (Fawcett, Seekins, Whang, Muiu, & Suarez de Balcazar, 1982). Concerns data from poverty families (Seekins & Fawcett, 1987), residents of low-income neighborhoods (Schriner & Fawcett, 1988), people with physical disabilities (Fawcett, Suarez de Balcazar, Whang-Ramos, Seekins, Bradford, & Mathews, 1988), or other client groups can shape collaborative relationships by helping to build a consensus about agendas for both research and action.

The *idea of problem,* used extensively in the behavior-analytic model, is another key concept in community research and action. When research is driven by issues defined by clients, rather than by those defined by the discipline, we have a greater chance of discovering variables that will contribute to actions that are acceptable to communities and outcomes that are valued by them.

A *problem* is a discrepancy between an actual and an ideal level of behavior and related community conditions that is labeled by communities of interest as important. Communities may label a situation as problematic because of one or more aspects of the behavior or condition, such as its frequency or duration. For example, frequency may be a problem if there is a discrepancy between actual and ideal numbers of low-income people registered to vote (Fawcett, Seekins, & Silber, 1988). For some clients, such as welfare rights organizers, the actual frequency may be too low. For others, including many incumbent elected officials, the condition may not be labeled as a problem, because avoiding an influx of new voters may be in their interest. Regardless of the kind of discrepancy, however, its legitimacy depends on its being labeled as problematic by true clients—those persons primarily affected by the behavior and related conditions in the community.

Problems are not reflected in community members alone. They may be seen in mediators or service providers, the community structure or system, or some combination of these. The problem of unemployment, for example, may be identified both in community members who are out of work and in the community's employment opportunities that show a discrepancy between the number of available jobs paying a just wage and the number of people (whether skilled or unskilled in job finding) seeking such employment.

Problem statements need not be "victim blaming" (Ryan, 1971). Functional problem statements acknowledge discrepancies in dimensions valued by those affected: They do not convey the notion that people are "bags of deficits." Rather than deflecting attention away from system variables, such problem statements can give primacy to client issues rather than to concerns of the discipline.

The question of *what levels of problems should be studied and acted upon* relates to the distinction between first- and second-order changes. First-order changes are those within a context that itself remains unchanged; second-order changes are those in the basic systems in which wealth and power are distributed (Watzlawick, Weakland, & Fisch, 1974). Perhaps for pragmatic reasons, we have been slow to shift research and action to higher-order targets within the ecosystem, for example, from welfare clients to decision makers. When we do so, community research and action can be extended to new independent and dependent variables, such as the effects of voter-registration campaigns on resource allocations to poverty programs or the effects of divestment by international corporations on compliance with human rights practices.

The difficulty in effecting any change, however, especially second-order change, suggests the importance of another concept, the *strategy of seeking small wins* (Weick, 1984). Too often, community psychologists dismiss such controllable outcomes, justifying inaction with the assertion that modest changes fail to affect the broader context and system. Small wins are important, however, because they have detectable consequences that help maintain social action over the long haul. Although we should continue to challenge each other to effect systemic change, we must also discover how to detect and credit those modest approximations of goal attainment known as small wins.

These choices of goals, clients, and levels cannot be separated from a consideration of the *values of researcher-collaborators*. Those of us who are predisposed to the value of freedom, for instance, will be more likely to design social interventions to affect the number and range of choices available to consumers. By contrast, those who are particularly sensitive to injustice will be more likely to select such problems as inequality of opportunity or inequity in the distribution of resources among potential beneficiaries.

The kinds of community conditions that we value and our choices of targets for research and action are, in turn, affected by the *broader context of research and action*. One feature of the broader context is the type of change model used (Rothman & Tropman, 1987). Models of change—whether prevention, empowerment, conflict organization, or community development—affect which discrepancies are targeted, the resources mobilized for action, and the timing of the intervention. Individual community change projects should be consistent with an overall model of social change.

A second important feature of the broader context is the likelihood of disapproval from powerful client audiences. Decision makers and power elites may decry social action components of research or even threaten the researchers and their institutions with retribution. My colleagues and I have described elsewhere separate incidents in which state legislators and local officials denounced research and action efforts directed toward them as "advocacy" or "lobbying" (Fawcett, Seekins, & Jason, 1987; Seekins, Maynard-Moody, & Fawcett, 1987). Yet it is possible to maintain scientific standards while generating and communicating knowledge that is likely to benefit clients (Coleman, 1972). Taking sides and bearing witness to the truth are necessary to transform research knowledge into community change (Price, 1988). However, this is usually done *despite* the broader context, which does little to support the tight coupling of community research and action.

A final aspect of the broader context to be considered is the control exerted by client audiences. Those audiences that provide clearer standards and more powerful consequences exert greater control over our research and action. Academic disciplines, such as psychology, promulgate standards suggesting that it is proper for researchers to determine what questions to ask, what measures and interventions to use, and whether the effects are significant. Until academic disciplines are held accountable to client audiences for their contributions to improvement as well as to understanding, we should expect continued emphasis on methodological rigor, rather than on societal benefit, and promulgation and enforced compliance with these standards through systems of graduate training and peer reviewing in professional journals. Professional journals in Community Psychology, with their emphasis on description rather than on action, place a higher value on whether theoretical relationships of interest to the discipline are demonstrated than on whether the community studied actually benefited from the research (Walsh, 1987b). More fundamentally, the view that problem solving is not actually science further delimits opportunities to contribute to society through currently conceived modes of community research and action.

EMERGING STANDARDS FOR COMMUNITY RESEARCH AND ACTION

Articulating standards for community research and action could contribute to the solution of puzzles confronted in this endeavor. The 10 standards outlined in this section reflect the complementary contributions of traditional and behavior-analytic paradigms and may be useful in charting a more functional course for the field.

Standards for Collaborative Relationships

A proposed standard for establishing collaborative relationships between researchers and those who are studied attempts to characterize an important tradition in anthropology and ethnography (e.g., Agar, 1980), community organization (Rothman & Tropman, 1987), and community psychology (e.g., Chavis et al., 1983; Kelly, 1986a; and Serrano-García, 1984). This standard is consistent with the constitutional ideal of the consent of the governed (Adler, 1987)—an idea that calls for a reciprocal relationship between citizens (clients) and public servants (researchers).

Standard 1. Community researchers should form collaborative relationships with the participants with whom they do research. Several questions may help assess the quality of the collaboration: (a) To what extent is the "emic" (native or insiders') view of the community and its goals represented in the research goals along with the researchers' view? (b) To what degree is the community's influence evident in the identification or choice of new research questions that are not suggested by either the discipline or the researchers' past choices of topics? (c) Does the method system require that the researcher become sufficiently knowledgeable about local ways by participating in activities of local origin—not just research activities—before, during, and after data collection? (d) If an intervention is used, is it designed, adapted, and implemented in collaboration with participants? (e) To what extent is the work responsive to initiatives from the community—does it encourage such initiatives, and do community members describe the research and action goals as their own?

Standards for Research Goals and Methodology

Emerging standards for research goals and methods reflect contributions from the methodology of quasi-experimentation (Cook & Campbell, 1979), applied behavioral research (Baer, Wolf, & Risley, 1968, 1987), social validation (Wolf, 1978), and the values and traditions of community psychology (e.g., Heller, Price, Reinharz, Riger, & Wandersman, 1984; Rappaport, 1977).

Standard 2. Descriptive community research should provide information about relationships between environmental events, behaviors presumed relevant to community functioning, and related outcomes valued by communities. Some key questions help evaluate the contribution of descriptive research: (a) To what degree are the strengths and problems of people in communities given priority over questions of concern merely to the discipline? (b) How adequately does the research contribute to our understanding of naturally occurring aspects of the setting and of participants' behavior over time? (c) Does the research contribute knowledge about what naturally occurring changes in behavior or environmental events, such as development of competence or changes in laws, bring about and maintain changes in the behavior and the related community conditions identified as problems? (d) To what extent does the research document the full variety of functional arrangements that enable or facilitate attainment of individual and community goals?

Standard 3. Experimental community research should provide information on the effects of modifiable and sustainable environmental events on behaviors and outcomes of interest, on the generality and maintenance of the effects, and on the social importance and appropriateness of the research and action. Using within- and between-group designs and appropriate analytical methods, experimental research should yield valid and reliable answers to these questions: (a) Is there evidence of internal validity—that is, does the experimental design rule out other plausible explanations of the effects? (To what extent does the independent variable produce changes in the behaviors and processes labeled as the problem or in the outcomes, such as productivity or incidence of disease, that are labeled as the problem?) (b) Is there "subject generality?" (To what degree do the effects generalize across participants?) (c) Is there stimulus generalization or setting generality? (To what extent do the effects generalize across conditions, settings, or stimulus situations?) (d) Is there "maintenance" of effects? (Over what duration are the effects sustained?) (e) Is there evidence of response generalization? (That is, are other behaviors and outcomes also affected?) (To what degree do the effects generalize to other important behaviors and outcomes?) (f) Is there social validity? (To what extent are the goals and target behaviors socially important from the perspective of clients? Are the procedures used in this social intervention acceptable to participants? Are the effects of the intervention socially significant according to clients? Do the effects lead people to say that the problem is solved or the goal is attained?) (g) Are there side effects? (What are the unintended consequences, both positive and negative, of the intervention suggested by follow-up observations of the setting and by interviews with participants?)

Standard 4. The chosen setting, participants, and research measures should be appropriate to the community problem under investigation. To judge the validity of settings, participants, and measures, the following questions are useful: (a) Are the participants studied in their own natural settings, and to what extent are the normal, valued features of the context undisturbed as a result of the research? (b) If the goal of the research is to solve a problem, do the chosen participants and setting actually experience the problem at a level that is socially important? (They should not be chosen for the convenience of the investigators.) (c) Is there sufficient evidence that the participants in the setting to be observed are the ones in whom the problem actually resides, or is the locus of the problem at a different level? (Perhaps the problem is with administrators, service providers, or decision makers, and not with the targets, who are insufficiently empowered to avoid the research.) (d) If the problem is with a behavior or community condition, is that condition measured, and not a rating, verbal statement, or some other proxy for the issue of interest? (e) If questionnaires are used, are additional direct measures of the behavior and conditions related to the problem also taken, to avoid exclusive reliance on proxy measures?

Standard 5. The measurement of dependent variables must be replicable by typically trained readers of community research reports, and chosen measures should attempt to capture the dynamic and transactional nature of the interaction between behavior and the environment. Evaluative questions for judging the reliability and sensitivity of the measurement system include: (a) To what extent can other researchers implement the behavioral observation systems (i.e., behavioral definitions, observer scoring instructions), rating scales, and other assessment instruments used to collect dependent measures? (b) Can the observers, scoring simultaneously but independently, produce satisfactorily high levels of interobserver agreement using the measurement system? (c) In addition to measures of the behavior of people in communities, does the research include measures of events in the environment? (d) Does the research provide measures of transactions between people's behavior and events in the environment? (Measures of mutual aid, for example, would presumably indicate both disclosures of need and others' provision of aid.) (e) To what degree are the measures sensitive to variations in the phenomena over time, in ways such as those provided by time series designs and longitudinal studies? (f) Do the measures convey the influence of behavior on environments as well as the influence of environmental events on behavior? (Evaluations of empowerment efforts, for example, would perhaps show evidence that the intervention affected the participants' behavior and that participants, in turn, effected changes in specific features of their environment.) (g) Are qualitative data, such as those gathered in ethnographic or structured interviews, used to complement knowledge gained through quantitative research?

Standards for Intervention and Dissemination

Standards for community intervention and dissemination of social innovations are drawn from the literatures on behavioral principles and procedures (e.g., Zeiler, 1978) and strategies for designing and disseminating social interventions (e.g., Seekins & Fawcett, 1984).

Standard 6. Community interventions should be replicable by typically trained implementors and sustainable with local resources. Questions helpful in evaluating social interventions include: (a) To what extent can other community researchers and typical collaborators implement the procedures (i.e., instructions, prompts, reinforcement, environmental design changes) that make up the social intervention? (b) To what degree are the effects on the behaviors and outcomes of interest replicable in different communities, including those with similar goals but different resources and different participant and setting characteristics? (c) Does the social intervention rely sufficiently on local resources (i.e., people, setting features, money, equipment, and events), and is the intervention maintained by the local community? (d) To what extent do the effects of the social intervention continue after the researchers' departure?

Standard 7. Community action should occur at the level of change and timing likely to optimize beneficial outcomes. The choice of level should reflect an understanding of these questions: (a) What behaviors (by whom and under what conditions) produce and maintain the community conditions that are labeled as the problem of interest? (b) What practical variables (implemented by whom and under what conditions) produce favorable changes in the behaviors and conditions that are labeled as problems? (c) What particular changes in behavior and outcomes (of whom and under what conditions) optimize desired changes in other behaviors and outcomes related to the problem or goal? (d) What timing and situational features represent the most favorable circumstances for community action?

Standard 8. Researchers should develop a capacity to disseminate the effective social interventions they develop and provide training and technical assistance to change agents. Evaluative questions regarding dissemination, technical assistance, and training include the following: (a) How will standards for using the social intervention be established, and consequences for meeting them be arranged, so that long-term fidelity to the model and resulting effectiveness are more likely? (b) How will adaptations of the social intervention or its components be arranged, so that the intervention will fit local conditions while it maintains similar levels of effectiveness? (c) How will the price (in time and money) be set so that the social intervention will be affordable by typical adopters? (d) How will technical assistance and support systems be used to embed the social intervention in the natural environment after the departure of the disseminators? (e) How will training be provided to increase the number and quality of change agents available in local communities?

Standards for Advocacy and Community Change

Standards for communicating the results of community research and action and assessing its impact reflect ideas for combining science and advocacy (Coleman, 1972; Price, 1988), the ethics of social intervention (Warwick & Kelman, 1976), and evolving models of prevention (Price, Cowen, Lorion, & Ramos-McKay, 1988) and empowerment (Fawcett et al., 1984; Rappaport, 1981, 1987).

Standard 9. Results of community research and action must be communicated openly and effectively to clients, implementors, and purchasers of social interventions, decision makers and, when appropriate, to the broader public. Communication efforts should reflect several concerns: (a) To what degree are the results conveyed to community member-collaborators in a way that is demystifying, comprehensible, and contributory to understanding and future action? (b) Are the results communicated to disciplinary audiences so as to permit an assessment of the adequacy of the method system and results and so as to contribute to the field's understanding of communities and their capacities for change? (c) Are the results communicated to decision makers in a way that contributes to substantive actions on behalf of people living in the contexts that are studied? (d) To what extent are the results framed to minimize their being used to justify the blaming of relatively marginal and unempowered people for their problems in living? (e) To what extent are the results communicated openly, even when at least some of the clients, researchers, collaborators, purchasers, or decision makers may not benefit from open communication? (See Price, 1988, for a consideration of some of the serious dilemmas of truth-telling.) (f) Does communication also flow from relevant audiences to researchers, providing the clients' perspectives on what was important about the research and action?

Standard 10. Community research and action projects should contribute to understanding and *change, especially that which fosters prevention of problems in living and empowerment of people of marginal status.* Questions useful in assessing the contribution to community change include the following: (a) Who are the clients? How much, and in what ways, does each benefit from the research and action? (b) In particular, to what extent are the lives of clients of relatively marginal and disempowered status improved by the research and action? (c) How adequately does the social intervention increase the number of people, events, and settings available to facilitate attainment of community goals? (d) To what degree does the intervention enhance the capacities of existing resources to meet individual and group goals? (e) To what extent are the small wins or improvements consistent with a larger plan or model for social change?

CLOSING COMMENTARY

These 10 standards, emerging from a synthesis of research paradigms, identify promising ideals for the field. As modified to face a changing array of puzzles, they suggest guidelines for planning and evaluating our work. Should these (or other) standards be adopted, perhaps new or modified arrangements will be necessary to facilitate their attainment. These may include new undergraduate training programs in community research and action, adjustments in existing graduate training and peer-reviewing criteria, new journals devoted to the integration of research and action, and revised journal policies setting a percentage of journal space for such work. Other promising approaches include creating interdisciplinary institutes for change agents, expanding the labor market for practitioners of the model, and establishing and enhancing rewards and recognition for community research and action (see Keys, 1988, for a discussion of strategies for supporting community research in the public interest).

It is in the fusion of research and action that community psychology can best fulfill its dream. We can achieve distinction by serving as a model of science in the public interest. As we attempt to live up to these ideals, we might be guided by Martin Luther King's (1968) call for leaders in service to higher values:

> Yes, if you want to say that I was a drum major, say that I was a drum major for justice; say that I was a drum major for peace; I was a drum major for righteousness. And all of the other shallow things will not matter.

. . . I just want to be there in love and in justice and in truth and in commitment to others, so that we can make of this old world a new world.

Perhaps future historians will use similar values and standards to judge community psychology's contributions to understanding and improvement. Should they do so, and should the field measure up, this old world will be a little better off for our presence.

CHAPTER 8

CRITERIA OF EXCELLENCE I. MODELS FOR ADVENTURESOME RESEARCH IN COMMUNITY PSYCHOLOGY:
COMMONALITIES, DILEMMAS, AND FUTURE DIRECTIONS

DAVID S. GLENWICK, KENNETH HELLER, JEAN ANN LINNEY, AND
KENNETH I. PARGAMENT

Chapters 3 through 5 have presented a range of perspectives—ecological, developmental, organizational, empowerment, and behavior-analytic—on researching phenomena of interest in community psychology. Despite their differing emphases, these perspectives may possess more in common than one might initially assume. These commonalities suggest what the standards could be for valid and useful theories, or at least perspectives, in community psychology.

In this chapter, we shall first outline these commonalities and then consider some of the dilemmas or tensions that are raised by the various perspectives. We will then suggest future directions for the use of theory to guide community psychology research. Finally, we will attempt to place in context the issue of theory and adventuresome research in community psychology by exploring two influential forces, one intellectual—the postmodernist movement, and the other organizational—the academic psychology department.

COMMONALITIES

1. Context and Ecology

Neither the research process itself nor the subject of a research investigation occurs in a social vacuum. Contextual forces shape both the phenomena of interest and the process of studying those phenomena. These forces may be context-specific, cultural, and/or temporal. The notion of context is of obvious centrality to the ecological perspective. We come to understand by observing persons or groups within the systems or contexts within which they function. The manner in which roles, social norms, and resources are created and their interdependence with particular persons and settings form the basis of knowledge of those persons and settings. Although context may be less of a core construct for some of the other perspectives, it is relevant to them as well.

2. The Reciprocal Relationship Between the Individual and the Social System or Environment

Awareness of context points to the importance of the relationship between the individual and his or her environment. The specific terms used by the authors of the preceding chapters to describe the nature of this relationship—*transactional, mutual, reciprocal*—may differ. What they share, however, is the idea that persons and settings engage in a multidirectional influence process among one another. For Rappaport, for example (see Chapter 6), the process of empowerment is embedded in relationships among people, organizations, and communities. Because this transactional process is a continuous and synergistic one, observes Lorion (see Chapter 4), both individual and environmental processes need to be monitored simultaneously; for the developmentalist, then, intervention alters one aspect of the situation to influence both processes in a desired direction.

These approaches all recognize that not only persons but also communities are "involved in a transactional relationship with the broader social and cultural context," as Lorion points out (see chapter 4). Such recognition highlights the need for multilevel analyses of phenomena, because the various levels at which each phenomenon may be studied (person, group, organization, community, and society) are related to and influence each other over time. Shifting from a focus on the individual or even on the individual–environment transaction to a focus on the transaction among several levels assists us in uncovering what Seidman (1988) referred to as *social regularities*—predictable patterns of social relations—which may then be targeted for intervention. Multilevel analysis can facilitate the investigation of higher-order targets in the ecosystem (e.g., decision makers), as urged

---

The order of authorship for the second, third, and fourth authors is alphabetical because each contributed equally.

by Fawcett (see Chapter 7), and has considerable potential for expanding the scope of change in behavior–environment relations at the levels of individuals, settings, and broader social systems.

3. The Temporal Dimension: The Role of Time and Process

Transactional relationships, by definition, occur over time. Although an inherent central focus of the developmental perspective, change patterns are crucial to the other perspectives as well. Most of us would probably agree that these processes are "identifiable, measurable, and, ideally, controllable lawful processes" (see Chapter 4). Both growth and dysfunction are evolutionary phenomena. Thus, from Rappaport's perspective, empowerment is a process occurring over time (see Chapter 6). Similarly, Kingry-Westergaard and Kelly, as ecological theorists, advocate longitudinal study of people, organizations, and policies in order to elucidate the process by which roles, norms, and resources are created (see Chapter 3). Sensitivity to variation in phenomena over time is also evidenced by the behavior analyst's fondness for time-series designs (see Chapter 7).

Attention to processes and the temporal dimension helps us conceptualize how we might carry out prevention research. That is, by manipulating such processes we can influence the development of both maladaptive and adaptive behaviors.

4. The Directedness of Events

Consideration of time and process sharpens our recognition that, as the behavior analyst stresses (see Chapter 7), both past and current events (i.e., one's early history of rewards and present contingencies of reinforcement) affect behavior, and that, as the developmentalist (see Chapter 4) highlights, there is a continuity in performance over the life span. Such continuity applies to the development of groups, organizations, and communities, as well as to individuals. Thus, the directedness of phenomena refers to their nonrandom quality. It is this nonrandomness that enables us to seek regularities in relationships and to attempt to modify them in desirable, specified directions.

5. Knowledge as a Constructed Phenomenon

Just as the phenomena that we study cannot be understood without consideration of their context, so too is the research process itself greatly determined by the context in which it unfolds. Discovery does not occur in a vacuum and does not result from pure, detached objectivity; rather, the act of knowing is a constructive and evolutionary process (see Chapter 3), dependent on the investigator's frame of reference and the context of activities constituting the research (see Chapter 5).

6. The Interrelationships Between the Observer and the Observed

Recognition of the interpersonal nature of the research process brings us to a new perspective on the roles of, and the relationship between, the observer and the observed. Traditionally this relationship has been conceptualized as one between a detached expert and a subject or subjects, the former being the party who formulates the questions of interest, decides on the research procedure, and analyzes and interprets the findings. The perspectives in the preceding chapters argue for a radically different relationship, in which the parties function as collaborators in a mutual-influence process. Thus, the scientist, the "targets" of the intervention, and the consumers of the research all become involved participants in the process. The constructed meaning of a phenomenon depends on the reciprocal relationships existing between the observer and the observed.

In a nonexploitive, collaborative relationship, there is a sharing of presuppositions, information, resources, results, and benefits by all parties throughout the research process. Because of this sharing, which incorporates stakeholders' perspectives on the phenomena of interest, more contextually relevant questions may be asked, more sensitive research methods chosen, and improved data interpretation arrived at, as Fawcett (see Chapter 7) remarks. The result, we may conclude with Fawcett, is better and richer science.

7. Subjectivity and the Perspective of "Subordinates"

A further implication of obtaining the perspective of "subordinates" (i.e., the "targets" or "subjects" of our research) is the legitimization of subjective experience. As Kingry-Westergaard and Kelly (see Chapter 3) state, the validity of our theoretical propositions will depend, in part, on the meaning of these propositions in the actual experience of community members. What is the context of the lives of the unempowered at the bottom of the organizational heap (see Chapter 5)? What resources and choices do they perceive themselves as having? Interestingly, even the behavior-analytic paradigm, frequently represented as the epitome of the traditional approach to research, has begun, in the past decade, to attend to subjective experience, through its inclusion of social validity (i.e., "subjects'" and consumers' perceptions regarding the goals, procedures, and results of the intervention) in the research process.

8. Empowerment as a Unifying Goal

If we view the research process as a collaborative one in which the role of subjective experience is explicitly acknowledged and positively regarded, then the impossibility of value- or goal-free research becomes apparent. The concept of empowerment directs us to concentrate on the resources in our society—to define and to measure access to them and to attend to how they are unequally distributed across constituencies. Consonant with this position, the ecological perspective examines roles and norms not as ends in themselves but with respect to their part in the activation and dispersion or concentration of resources. Fawcett, from the behavior-analytic perspective (see Chapter 7), echoes the belief that community psychology should serve to empower those with whom we work. As the behavior-analyst might put it, how are the reinforcers in our society apportioned, and who controls the opportunities to obtain them?

One may take issue with empowerment as *the* unifying goal for community psychology research (see the sixth dilemma below). Consideration of it, however, does help to remind us that values and goals, implicitly or explicitly, are intrinsic to and have a shaping role in the research process.

9. Reliability of Observations

Recognition of the part that subjective experience plays in all research should not cause us to dismiss the desirability of also attempting to obtain observations that are reliable. With its concentration on overt behavior and observable outcomes, the behavior-analytic perspective's stress on reliable measurement probably has been one of its greatest strengths. Attention to reliability of observation may complement the more phenomenological, experiential approach discussed above. The use of both approaches may result in the broader, more integrative approach advocated by Fawcett (see Chapter 7), in which reliable observations, introspection, and ecological validity (i.e., awareness of contextual factors) all contribute to the construction of meaning.

These nine themes are strands running through all the perspectives described in the previous five chapters. They suggest that there is, indeed, a fair degree of overlap in the underlying assumptions and postulates of these perspectives. These commonalities should help guide us in developing (a) the standards for evaluating the adequacy of models in community psychology and (b) the qualities that a heuristically valuable model is likely to possess.

DILEMMAS AND TENSIONS

Commonalities notwithstanding, consideration of the various perspectives or models leads to the realization that there are a number of problems, or tensions, that we must address in grappling with the question of the nature of the relationship between theory and research in community psychology.

1. The Limited Applicability of Our Theories

We need to ask ourselves whether we need one paradigmatic theory (is one possible?) or several theories of community and community change, and how close we are to formulating it or them. The major current perspectives differ considerably in their emphases, despite their shared features. Some (e.g., empowerment) stress particular goals or values rather than how the goals come to be understood and accomplished, some (e.g., ecological) point to research variables and processes of importance to community researchers, and some (e.g., behavioral, organizational, developmental) propose predetermined metaframeworks that provide methodologies by which theories of community phenomena might be constructed. In addition, the perspectives are at different explanatory levels: Empowerment and ecology (i.e., context) may be thought of as metaconcepts, capable of informing a variety of substantive approaches, whereas the behavioral, developmental, and organizational views are more substantive perspectives.

Another limitation is that our research results are typically not directly generalizable to other settings, conditions, and times, by design. This limitation will impede theory-building in the traditional sense of piece-by-piece knowledge verification.

Thus, it appears that, at present and for the foreseeable future, we may regard community psychology theory as being in a preparadigmatic state (Kuhn, 1970). None of the current perspectives allows answers to the major questions of the field in a manner clearly superior to other perspectives. The best that we may hope for are "approaches," "models," or "minitheories" that provide us with orienting perspectives—places and ways to look in order to understand selected phenomena—and that contribute to the delineation of the variables of interest. Such a view is consistent with Cronbach's (1975) statement that, in psychology as a whole, the days of grand, overarching theories may be behind us and that theories with more limited ambitions, explanatory power, and generalizability may prove more useful in directing and interpreting psychological research.

2. The Tension Between Our Commitment to Diversity/ Relativism and to Theory Testing

A dedication to tolerance and diversity has been among community psychology's hallmark values. However, our commitment to these can hinder us in trying to push each perspective as far as it will go and testing its limits (see the second item in Future Directions below, as well as Shadish's discussion in Chapter 2 of descriptive vs. prescriptive values).

3. The Tension Between Ethnography and Intervention

As community psychologists, we think that it is important to describe phenomena of interest because we see behavior in a social context, and because understanding that social context is important. At the same time, part of our mission as community psychologists is to take action and to be helpful to others. Studying a phenomenon and not acting, that is, not intervening, can be a "cop-out." On the other hand, while doing informs, doing before one is informed imposes costs as well.

On this dimension, the five perspectives in the preceding chapters evidence somewhat divergent emphases. For example, the ecological and developmental perspectives appear to emphasize ethnography, that is, description (although certainly not to the exclusion of intervention), whereas the behavior-analytic and empowerment perspectives seem to concentrate more on intervention. These emphases can produce different kinds of understanding, for example, conceptual understanding (the ecological perspective) as opposed to instrumental understanding (the behavior-analytic perspective), to use Shadish's terminology (see Chapter 2).

4. The Dilemma of "Slices" and "Scans"

Looking at behavior in "slices"—our traditional cross-sectional method—allows us to look with experimental control. Taking "scans," a longitudinal approach, allows us to look more at behaviors in a social context. Both strategies have costs and benefits. Carrying out experimental research probably gives us a clearer grasp, at least of the slice of behavior that is examined, and permits us to do more in terms of actually confirming our knowledge. But to study the slice without the context of the scan will very likely result in a sterile understanding.

Furthermore, we have to recognize that there are values embedded in both of these approaches. Our community constituencies and collaborators may hold different perspectives and different values on this issue than we do, perhaps wanting us to be experts who help them present the best researchable case (be it slices or scans) for their particular point of view.

5. The Dilemma of Collaboration

Collaboration also presents difficulties. Although earlier in the chapter we outlined the virtues of collaboration with community members, there are costs and tensions involved in such collaboration. When do you collaborate—at what point in time? How do you set up the collaborative process and maintain it? If, as a result of the mutual influence process described above, you keep changing the nature of the research as you are collaborating, at some point you will cloud the lens through which you are looking at behavior. Thus, collaboration may entail a trade-off, with a loss of clarity and reliability perhaps being the price of increased responsiveness to the community.

6. The Values Dilemma

Different perspectives, because of their different underlying values, may lead to different definitions of the good or ideal life and to different strategies for how to achieve it. The value orientation highlighted in the present volume has been that of empowerment. However, it should be noted that there are probably other valid values and goals, such as fraternity, sense of community, liberty, and equality of opportunity. Not only theoretical perspectives, but also various community constituencies may differ in the primary values that impel their interests and activities.

These problems are illustrative of the issues confronting the community psychology researcher who would be guided by theory. Obviously they do not admit of easy resolution, and community psychologists may reasonably differ with respect to which side of the scale they choose to put their weight on. Moreover, the answers arrived at by the individual researcher are likely to vary depending on the particular approach that is adopted.

FUTURE DIRECTIONS

Up to this point, our discussion has focused on the present state of the relationship between theory and research in community psychology. In this section we offer some directions that conceptual and empirical work might profitably take in the future.

1. Draw on the Strengths of the Various Alternative Perspectives

Both for community psychology as a discipline and for the individual researcher, designing research that incorporates the concepts of several perspectives may be a step toward building multiple viewpoints into our work and thereby improving its quality. Because each perspective has its own pluses and minuses and unique contextual focus, each can help us learn different things about a given phenomenon. Even when operating from a dominant perspective, our willingness to borrow from other perspectives can enhance a study's comprehensiveness and sophistication and aid in addressing social problems more effectively. For example, a behavior analyst might bring in the transactional approach of the developmental perspective in examining person–environment influences and exchanges.

As discussed earlier, the probability is not high that any grand, paradigm-like theory will gain ascendance in community psychology. If this were to come to pass, however, it would probably come from hybrid, multiperspective research and be an amalgam of the key constructs and ideas of several perspectives.

2. Carry the Implications of Each Perspective as far as They Will Go

In contrast to the previous recommendation, it can be argued that a multiapproach strategy obscures the differences that exist among perspectives and that the explanatory power of each can be truly determined only by testing its limits. Thus, an alternative to the multiperspective orientation is for each perspective's adherents to lay out clearly that perspective's basic assumptions and postulates and see where they lead. Researchers operating from this stance could start with the phenomenon of interest and think about how their perspective could be applied to its investigation. The process is a bidirectional one. That is, the phenomenon of interest, and the questions asked about it, will very likely influence which perspectives prove to be most appropriate for it. At the same time, the perspectives held will greatly determine the choice of questions about a given phenomenon and the form that these questions take.

It is hoped that adopting this strategy will lead to exemplars that illustrate upon which phenomena each perspective is good at shedding light. For instance, in Chapter 4 in this volume, Lorion describes how a developmental perspective, through the concept of transactions, may be useful in making predictions concerning high-risk kindergartenners; and, in Chapter 5, Riger demonstrates how, with the organizational perspective, one can examine such target groups as tenant organizations and ex-hospitalized patients.

While this approach to theory-driven research will capitalize on each perspective's distinct virtues, it will probably cause us to discover that no one perspective possesses sufficient explanatory power. The consequence would then be either (a) the coexistence of several models that are differentially helpful in gaining knowledge about a variety of problems or (b) a hybrid model or theory.

3. Construct and Apply Additional Models

Though dominant today, the five perspectives upon which this volume focuses should not be regarded as exhausting the realm of possible theoretical models. Greater attention to other proposed models, such as historical and cultural analyses (Levine, 1981, and Sarason, 1982a, 1982b) and Marxist perspectives, is warranted, and the building and application of new models should be encouraged as well.

4. Draw on Our Community-Based Research and Practice To Assist in Model Construction

Community psychologists, through direct interactions with community organizations and social systems, have accumulated a wealth of experience and data. We need to consider the implications of this phenomenological and empirical knowledge for the theories that we build. Everyone doing community psychology operates from an implicit theory; we should use our research and practice to inform our models.

5. Incorporate Both Objective and Subjective Approaches in Our Research

Traditional, objective research may be thought of as a narrow, funneling-down process, in which each subsequent investigation is designed to play out the implications of previous research. It is a winnowing process, intended to isolate singular causal relationships. This approach can be complemented by a more subjective, context-based one that might be called a *funneling-up* process, in which each subsequent investigation contributes a new layer of understanding by adding variables or a new context. Community psychology would thus benefit from recognizing that connection and empathy are valid modes of knowing and that both subjective and objective approaches are valuable and can be integrated in our research.

6. Encourage Collaboration Between Community Psychology Researchers and the Participants or Community Constituents of Our Research

Collaborative research constantly tests our ideas by moving back and forth between the researcher's and the participants' concepts and experiences. Taking this recommendation seriously should assist in ensuring that alternative perspectives are reflected in our research, because the choice of collaborators will strongly affect the perspectives that we acquire on a problem.

7. Incorporate Analyses of Individual–Environment Transactions Into Our Research

We must go beyond traditional linear, unidirectional analyses and explore the reciprocal, ongoing relationships that occur between persons and settings. There is also a need for a language that can describe such connections between individuals and their social systems. Organizational psychology has some potentially useful constructs in this respect (e.g., *roles, climate,* and *status*), as does family systems theory (e.g., *boundaries, homeostasis,* and *enmeshment–disengagement*).

8. Build Multilevel Analyses Into Our Research

Such research should aid both in understanding existing phenomena (i.e., descriptive research) and in conducting research on changes to social systems in which we examine how change at one level affects behavior at another level (see Chapter 11 by M. Shinn, for a detailed discussion of this topic).

9. Conduct More Descriptive Research

An overemphasis on experimental research could restrict community psychology's development by functionally blinding us to alternative ways of viewing and of making sense of phenomena. The difference is like that between the astronomer, who focuses on describing patterns and naturally occurring change, and the experimental physicist, who is concerned with manipulation, reductionism, and the isolation of critical variables. Community psychology needs not only "experimental physicists" but also "astronomers" who explore patterns of relationships and provide the material on which experimental studies may be based. This issue is closely related to the third dilemma noted above, namely the difficulty of choosing between ethnography and intervention.

CONTEXT OF THEORY AND RESEARCH IN COMMUNITY PSYCHOLOGY: POSTMODERNISM AND THE ACADEMIC PSYCHOLOGY DEPARTMENT

Having stressed the importance of context in understanding any phenomenon of interest, we should apply this concept to this chapter's own phenomenon of interest. In this section, therefore, we discuss the influence of two contextual factors on community psychology theory and research. One—postmodernism—provides a sympathetic backdrop for the development of adventuresome theory and research. The second—the academic psychology department—has the potential to hinder creative conceptualization and activity.

Postmodernism

The period since World War II has been marked by an intellectual and social current that has come to be known as *postmodernism*. Rather than a unified set of beliefs, the postmodern movement is "an attitude, a frame of mind . . . a way of seeing the world and acting within it" (Schrag, 1988, p. 2). Its principal features include "the plurality of narratives, the multiplicity of language games, the heterogeneity of social practices, and the diversity of forms of knowledge" (p. 2). As Schrag puts it,

> If you are postmodern, you will resist the urge to tell big stories. . . . You will consolidate your discourse into local rather than grand narratives. You will steer clear of unifying principles and overarching designs that purport to tell the whole truth . . . about all time and existence. You will be suspicious of unities, celebrate plurality, [and] remain sensitive to differences. (p. 2)

From this perspective, it becomes difficult, if not impossible, to arrive at a generally accepted paradigm within any field. Thus, within any field explored by postmoderns, a number of competing models coexist, created by the community of practicing scientists in that field.

It becomes apparent that the state of theory and research in community psychology is essentially similar to the issues confronting other fields of knowledge. Therefore, as we grapple with these issues, we would do well to be attentive to postmodernist thought in general and to consider its implications for our own discipline.

The Academic Psychology Department

Although the challenges facing community psychology, and our recommendations for addressing these challenges, seem to have an intrinsic compatibility with postmodernism, this may not, unfortunately, be true of community psychology's relationship with academic psychology departments. In such disciplines as philosophy, postmodernism has come to be regarded as a legitimate, accepted mode of conceptualizing and investigating problems. However, in the academic psychology department, current research practice appears grounded in a way of thinking—logical positivism—that antedates postmodernism. Its dominant attributes are familiar: (a) the experimental method as the only way of knowing; (b) an experimenter who studies "subjects"; (c) an environment that is typically controlled and artificially manipulated; (d) a process that is "objective" and seemingly value-free; and (e) a focus that is short-term and interested in a single, or very few, points in time.

Thus, although the issues and problems outlined here are in the postmodern intellectual mainstream, they have yet to be reflected in the philosophy of knowing that undergirds most research conducted in academic psychology departments. For this reason, our field, in addition to providing supports and opportunities for fostering imaginativeness in theory-building and research, would do well to forge alliances with other psychologists interested in applied questions and innovative methods and epistomologies (e.g., Bronfenbrenner, 1977, who writes from a developmental vantage point).

CONCLUSION

It is told that the writer Gertrude Stein, when faced with the impending passing of her friend Alice B. Toklas, inquired of the latter as she lay on her deathbed, "Alice, what is the answer?" Pausing for a moment, Alice is said to have looked up and replied, "Gertrude, what is the question?" To its credit, community psychology has begun to question itself regarding the adequacy of its models and the research deriving from, and contributing to, them. The questions that we ask, and how we proceed to answer them, will determine the course of research and theory in our discipline in the coming decade. Such a self-examination process entails intellectual and professional risks and uncertainties; but, after all, shouldn't adventuresome research demand adventuresome researchers?

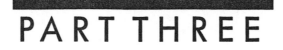

PART THREE

HYPOTHESIS GENERATION: FRAMING THE QUESTION

CHAPTER 9

PURSUING THE MEANING AND UTILITY OF SOCIAL REGULARITIES FOR COMMUNITY PSYCHOLOGY

EDWARD SEIDMAN

Throughout its history, Community Psychology has attached considerable importance to identifying its phenomena of interest (Glidewell, 1966; Rappaport, 1987; Seidman, 1988). Phenomena of interest stem from our world views and preferred theories. The specific form and nature of phenomena of interest are critical to the generation and framing of research questions and hypotheses consistent with our intentions and world views. Thus, to understand issues of hypothesis generation, we need to examine carefully the nature, form and origin of these phenomena; more importantly, appropriate measurement operations must follow, not precede, such an in-depth examination.

In my presidential address to APA's Division 27, I described *social regularities* as my recommended choice for Community Psychology's principal phenomenon of interest (Seidman, 1988). In order to unpack the construct of "social regularities," I begin this paper by offering a full examination of this construct's meaning and centrality to a theory of social intervention. Then I discuss the epistemological assumptions and premises that have hindered and may continue to hinder Community Psychology's exploration of social regularities. For brevity, I shall refer to these epistemological assumptions as biases. (It should be noted that whereas a bias may present a one-sided and somewhat distorted view, it also allows us to see some things more clearly.) Finally, I suggest initial ways for us to begin researching social regularities.

SOCIAL REGULARITIES

History

The construct of *social regularities* has antecedents in the history of Community Psychology as well as in earlier notions upon which Community Psychology was built. At Swampscott, the founders of Community Psychology defined the field by discussing the centrality of assessing "the reciprocal relationships between individuals and the social systems with which they interact" (Bennett et al., 1966, p. 7). What emerges from this emphasis is much more than a simple focus on community or individual variables. It is the reciprocal relationships, transactions, and interdependencies of individuals and social systems that represent the unique synthesis of community and psychology. This emphasis is similar to Lewin's assertion of the importance of the "relations between parts or elements" (1947/1951b, p. 192), Allport's "structurings of ongoings and events" (1962, p. 18), and Bateson's "connections that unite" (entities or elements that he referred to as the *relata,* or patterns of relations; 1972, 1979). Such dynamic constructs are transactional and explicitly antireductionistic (Altman & Rogoff, 1987).

We are not alone in striving to define our phenomena of interest as transactional and patterned. In fact, we are in step with the emergence of a field known as *structural analysis* in many of our sister social sciences. Also drawing upon general systems theory and cybernetics, structural analysis identifies the social exchange or relations among units—be they individuals, groups, corporations, nation-states, or other collectives—as the central phenomenon (Wellman & Berkowitz, 1988). This movement toward "structuralism" has also been apparent in the physical and biological sciences; for example, quantum physics defines the properties of parts by the interactions between them (Wellman & Berkowitz, 1988).

Definitions

A *social regularity* is a dynamic, temporal pattern of transactions (relations, connections, or linkages) between at least two units or entities that constitute a social system or setting. This definition includes four important components—units, settings, social nature, and temporal patterning.

Units, or *entities,* can be any meaningful role category, grouping of people, or organization(s), considered as a whole rather than by attributes. Some illustrative social units include the following: men and women; ethnic groups; management, rank and file, and consumers; patients and service delivery personnel; poor and wealthy people; and the judicial system and prisoners (as well as complex combinations of these).

Setting refers to a social system. The smallest is a dyad of two individuals, for example, a married couple. However, Community Psychology should not concern itself with social, or more precisely interpersonal, regularities within individual dyads and families. Instead, our focus of concern should be social regularities within settings larger than the family or between settings or systems.

The *Social nature,* or content or quality, of these regularities is obvious. Thus, as I have previously indicated, they "may center on clear-cut social relations, such as power, roles, status, participation, and communication, or on resources that are indirectly social, such as income, services, education, health, well-being, and leisure" (Seidman, 1988, p. 10).

Finally, *temporal patterning* is the constancy of social transactions over time—the essence of the regularity itself.

Meaning

A social regularity can be observed and described, but its salience can only be discerned by its functional linkage to persons. That is, the functional meaning of a social regularity ultimately derives from its predictable association with significant psychosocial outcomes. At a minimum, a social regularity constrains the possible psychosocial outcomes. This association occurs because a social regularity communicates and symbolizes information and meaning, whether actively perceived or not. For example, it is not surprising to find early adolescents becoming increasingly disaffiliated from school (the psychosocial outcome) at a time when they are developmentally capable of increased responsibility in the educational process, because the level of student participation in classroom learning does not increase commensurately with those capabilities. One illustration of this is that in most schools the ratio of questions asked by teacher to questions asked by students in classrooms remains similar from year to year. Thus, the pattern of transactions, or social regularity, is evidenced. Furthermore, neither the students nor the teachers need to be actively aware of this association for it to occur. This, like any other social regularity, represents a consistent pattern of transactions between the groups of actors over time. Thus, we can conceptualize social regularities as emergent processes related to psychosocial outcomes.

What is the time lag between the social regularity and associated psychosocial outcomes? Proximal association with psychosocial outcomes is less frequent or less apparent because psychosocial outcomes often take considerably more time to unfold; thus, this linkage is often presumed to be nonexistent, on the basis of cross-sectional data or the traditional, short-term follow-up design. Its occurrence is more accurately conceptualized and assessed distally (Seidman, 1987).[1] Pragmatically, however, researchers cannot wait for distal data on psychosocial outcomes to get a reading on the probable success of an intervention. We need not simply await the appearance of long-term psychosocial outcomes to assess the efficacy of an intervention; we can and should assess proximal changes in the social regularity itself. (For a more extensive discussion and illustration of this issue, see Seidman, 1987.)

---

[1]It should be recognized that *proximal* and *distal* are relative terms.

The Utility of Social Regularities for a Theory of Social Intervention

There are two imperative tasks in incorporating the concept of social regularities into a theory of social intervention. First, as suggested above, we need to identify the critical social regularities by means of their linkage to psychosocial outcomes. Second, once identified, a social regularity must be altered in order to affect the distal outcomes for a population of concern.

How can we alter a social regularity? Inherent in any social regularity is information about the structure of social transactions and its pattern over time. Here we can be guided by the emerging science of Chaos (Gleick, 1987), in which "sensitive dependence on initial conditions" has become the fundamental concept. This concept means that a slight alteration in initial conditions (in our field, the structure of social relations or of the conditions that influence them) can lead to the evolution of dramatically different temporal patterns of transactions and outcomes. Following these implications, we need to alter the initial conditions, or the structure of social relations, in order to ultimately influence psychosocial outcomes.

The exemplary work of Felner and his colleagues (Felner & Adan, 1988; Felner, Ginter, & Primavera, 1982) in developing, implementing, and evaluating the School Transitional Environment Project (STEP) illustrates the alteration of critical social regularities inherent in the transition to high school. Putting Sarason's writings (1972) into action, Felner observed that students face abrupt changes in peer networks and social ties to school staff upon entering high school. Immediately after the transition, many students no longer have a set of peers with whom they move through many of their classes, and they also have a different teacher in every class. There is little consistency in either the peers or adults whom students encounter from hour to hour.

Thus, the *initial conditions* that STEP endeavored to restructure included both the consistency of in-school peer networks and the students' ties to teachers and staff. Although these social regularities, or initial conditions, were not assessed, the intervention did alter the long-term psychosocial outcomes and opportunities for youth. For example, although the STEP program was only implemented during the first year of high school, only 21 percent of STEP participants dropped out of high school prior to graduation, in contrast to 43 percent of the control-group youth.

The work of Felner and his colleagues restructured the initial social conditions (structure), which, in turn, allowed a new social regularity and associated psychosocial outcomes to emerge at the level of the school. At the level of the classroom setting, Slavin (1983) and Aronson (1978) have developed a number of "games" to restructure the pattern of social transactions among students from one that fosters competition to one that fosters cooperation. The restructuring of this social regularity has consistently led to gains in academic performance, to improved social relations, particularly in the area of race relations, and to the acceptance of mainstreamed students' improved self-esteem.

UNITS OF ANALYSIS AND INHERENT BIASES

Why has it been so difficult to clearly identify—let alone assess and alter—social regularities? It is my contention that the biases inherent in a units-of-analysis approach have, often unwittingly, predetermined the nature of the phenomenon to be examined; this, in turn, has obstructed our pursuit of the meaning and utility of social regularities.

Psychology, even Community Psychology, has been dominated by the study of entities and of unidirectional and linear causal processes. Any entity, element, or "thing"—be it an individual, a population, an organization, or a state—can be characterized by its attributes or characteristics. By and large, the social sciences examine the attributes of entities. (We are not alone here; a similar approach dominated Newtonian physics.)

In psychology, individuals are most often described in terms of personal attributes (e.g., competency or aggression) that are independent of the specific environmental context. These attribute-centered assessment biases stem from a variety of unexamined premises, foremost of which are an individually oriented Western mindscape and the assumptions of an Aristotelian classification logic (Seidman, 1978, 1983, 1987, & 1988; Seidman & Rappaport, 1986). These unexamined premises predetermine the constructs and hypotheses that we investigate, the targets of intervention that we choose, and the locus of effects that we assess. To be consistent with the belief systems and rhetoric of community psychology, we must identify and use constructs that are transactional and recursive in nature, such as social regularities.

Different schemata for levels-of-analysis approaches have been put forward by Community Psychologists (Goodstein & Sandler, 1978; Murrell, 1973; Rappaport, 1977). To illustrate these attribute-centered biases, I shall use the individual, population, setting, and mesosystem framework that I recently described (Seidman, 1988). This framework highlights the differential biases by levels and the concomitant transition from entities and their attributes to social regularities as the phenomena of interest. Both are critical to understanding the target of intervention and the locus of effect (Seidman, 1987).

Individual and Population Units

Individual and population units of analysis identify entities as the phenomena of interest; the same set of epistemological assumptions undergirds both individual and population levels. The measurement of entities is most likely to be attribute-centered; thus, constructs like *anxiety* and *knowledge* are assessed. These are static phenomena. They lack the necessary temporal and transactional character of social regularities.

Even when it appears that social science research is going beyond the individual or population levels to extraindividual levels like an organization or community, the same biases determine the target of intervention and locus of effect; researchers remain locked into an examination of attributes of an organization or a community (e.g., its social climate). Despite the common conceptualization of organizations and communities as dynamic and systemic, the same biases result in populations being identified as the target of intervention and the locus of effect. Setting and mesosystem notions are intended to facilitate a shift (in basis) from attributes to social regularities, thus placing them center stage.

Setting and Mesosystem Units

Setting and mesosystem concepts suggest units that are dynamic and organizationally more complex, in contrast to the static attribute-centered foci of both individual and the commonly thought of extraindividual units of analysis. Settings and mesosystems are intentionally defined as such in order to highlight their social and transactional character and to ensure that they will not be mistakenly assessed using attribute-centered biases. These definitions make explicit the underlying epistemological shift from static, entity-centered constructs to dynamic social regularities. Social regularities are an emergent construct at both the setting and mesosystem levels. Settings focus on within-setting social regularities, and mesosystems focus on between-settings social regularities. Examples of settings include schools, human service agencies, and workplaces, whereas mesosystems are exemplified by policies that prescribe a pattern of transactions and procedures between settings.

The activity of settings and mesosystems takes the form of a dynamic and ongoing pattern or confluence of social transactions among its respective entities, even when its specific constituent entities change. Using the apt metaphor of a river to discuss racial discrimination, (an outstanding exemplar of a social regularity), Lewin wrote, "We are dealing with a process, which like a river, continuously changes its elements even if its velocity and direction remain the same" (1947/1951b, p. 202). In a social regularity, we are interested not only in the process, but also in the components that remain the same (velocity and direction).

At this point, it may be helpful to describe a social regularity at the setting level. Barker (1968) developed an intriguing operationalization of a social regularity at the setting level: the concept of manning or, in nonsexist terms, staffing. Staffing refers to the ratio of available roles in a setting to the number of setting inhabitants. Any setting has a finite number of roles, and, if there is a large number of setting inhabitants, the result is an overstaffed setting, where inhabitants find fewer roles and niches. In an understaffed setting on the other hand, inhabitants must occupy multiple roles in order to maintain the organization's goals and viability. Assessing the organizational attribute of size alone is insufficient to operationalize the social regularity. Size, by itself, is not a social regularity and stems from a different (attribute-centered) conceptual bias. Instead, a measure such as the ratio of roles to organizational size may capture better the true meaning of this social regularity. Whereas the number of members (entities) may change over time, the real question is whether the ratio of roles to size changes. If the ratio remains the same, it reflects a social regularity and may have important and predictable outcomes for its inhabitants in terms of satisfaction, continuation and performance, and psychological well-being. In other words, ultimately, the salience accorded to a setting's regularity—in this case, degree of staffing—stems from its functional relationship to the outcomes for its inhabitants.

Another example of social regularity may be unanticipated intervention effects. Linney (1986) evaluated a court-ordered desegregation plan, or mesosystem intervention. Ostensibly, the plan intended to restructure the social positions and transactions between Black and White students in a midwestern school system. Although students were brought together in the same classrooms and schools, the relative social positions of one group relative to the other seemed to be maintained within each school by new (and unplanned) means of segregation, such as disproportionate rates of referral of Black children to "special" classes. In effect, the "true" social regularity remained unchanged.

In sum, the attribute-centered biases inherent in individual and population units of analysis obscure our ability to identify, measure, and change transactional processes. Such objectives are only achievable if we work at the setting or mesosystem levels, where the biases are inherently social, transactional, and temporal in nature. Thus, when the gestalt to which our attention is directed is a setting or mesosystem (as opposed to an individual or population), social regularities can emerge into the foreground. Yet, as we have seen in the court-ordered desegregation example, clear identification and targeting of an apparent social regularity may not be sufficient to achieve the desired changes, either in the regularity or the ultimate psychosocial outcomes. If we do not target the salient social regularities, however, our interventions will be restricted to first-order changes (Watzlawick, Weakland, & Fisch, 1974).

RESEARCHING SOCIAL REGULARITIES

Up to this point, I have focused primarily on the conceptual structure or morphology of social regularities. In practice, our operationalizations are not always consistent with our theoretical specifications. This is the case even when our thinking is rooted in the soil of a setting or mesosystem. Thus, I now focus on the measurement of social regularities. At least three questions are critical: (a) How can social regularities be represented? (b) How can we assess their temporal pattern? (c) How do we determine their functional significance?

How Can Social Regularities Be Represented?

We must begin with some form of representation that is guided by a setting or mesosystem conceptualization. We hope that theory will dictate the specific form and content of the social regularity that we are attempting to discern, or at least point us in the right direction. The pattern of the regularity may, in fact, be its irregularity or its discontinuity. Using theory and extant knowledge, we must observe and describe the pattern over time.

As I have previously suggested, social regularities can be represented by "differences and ratios along one or more substantive dimensions. Differences occur *between* social units—groups, populations, or organizational entities; ratios represent a group or population in relation to a larger organizational unit" (Seidman, 1988, p. 9). In each case, a meaningful category of social actors is represented and, more important, it is represented in relation to another category of social actors. Each serves simultaneously as the context for the other. Unfortunately, such a static or cross-sectional representation of a social regularity runs the risk of ignoring the regularity itself, that is, its all-important emergent temporal pattern.

In What Ways Can the Temporal Pattern of a Social Regularity Be Assessed?

The simplest, most common, and potentially most fallible method of assessing temporal patterns is *inference* from cross-sectional analysis. That is, a social regularity, or more precisely a social relation, is measured at a single point in time. This approach resembles a single snapshot of the phenomenon, but is, nevertheless, conceptualized as a temporal regularity.

In some instances, this inferential process may not be a fallible operationalization. For example, one might assess the ratio of roles to students in a particular classroom—that is, its staffing—and infer that the ratio is a social regularity; this inference is fairly accurate, because the constituent parts of this ratio are unlikely to change much over the academic year. Moving to a mesosystem example, we find that the wealthiest 5 percent of the population earns over 19 percent of all income in this country, whereas the lowest 20 percent earns only 3.8 percent of all income. In this instance, the inference that this inequitable distribution of wealth is a social regularity is correct, because it can be substantiated by an examination of the annual census data over the past 20 years (U.S. Bureau of the Census, 1986). In both instances, the inference of a social regularity from the single snapshot would appear justified either on the basis of a logical analysis or other means of verification regarding its temporal patterning.

However, in a situation in which the relationship of the categories of social actors to each other is likely to evidence considerable irregularity from one point in time to another, the confidence placed in an inference from a single time measurement is questionable. For example, if, in assessing the regularity of police disposition decisions regarding juvenile offenders at weekly intervals, it is known that the decisions vary dramatically depending on the presiding judge of the week, an inference on the basis of a single week's measurement is unsound.

An alternative method of measuring social regularities is conceptually analogous to a series of snapshots of the relations among categories of social actors taken at repeated intervals. Operationally, a repeated series of difference or ratio scores, as described above, could be used. In a similar vein, within-group relative position or standing could index a social regularity by calculating a series of z scores over time.

Both the total span of time required and the particular intervals at which each snapshot is to be taken are critical to capture the nature of any particular social regularity accurately. Each social regularity is likely to have a rhythm of its own, and it may be difficult to anticipate the correct measurement intervals for an emergent temporal pattern. In fact, the effect may appear chaotic until the pattern emerges, as suggested by Chaos theory (Gleick, 1987). More frequent measurement may not be an effective antidote, because the salient phenomena may not always be observable. In sum, the span and time of repeated observations must be tailored to the particular social regularity of interest. To inform and guide these measurement operations, there is no substitute for good theory and prior knowledge. Only then will a series of snapshots increase our likelihood of capturing the emergent temporal pattern.

The last method of measuring social regularities resembles a film that requires continuous monitoring or recording. Of course, this is the most costly, difficult, and impractical method. Yet a "filmed record" is likely to be extremely accurate and reliable in capturing the social regularity if the particular social regularity is continuously observable. This mode of assessment, like the series of continuous snapshots, is dependent on monitoring the correct phenomenon for the appropriate time interval.

How Do We Determine the Functional Significance of a Social Regularity?

Ultimately, any social regularity is only meaningful to the degree that it is related at least distally to the lives of persons, in the cognitive, emotional, or behavioral domain (Seidman, 1987). The empirical relationships between a social regularity and individual well-being must be examined, of course, with the appropriate time lag. Again, in determining the "appropriate" time lag, there is no substitute for good theory or prior knowledge. It should also be realized that more than one social regularity may serve, predictably, the same function distally for the affected persons; this is analogous to the concept of multiplicity in developmental theory.

CONCLUSIONS AND IMPLICATIONS

A genuine Community Psychology must (a) examine the biases undergirding both our Western patterns of thought and our scientific theories, (b) strive to identify and target salient social regularities, and (c) with equal vigilance choose measurement operations that are congruent with our intentions. If we continue to think and work primarily at the individual and population levels, we are unlikely either to expand the needed generative research base or to identify the appropriate targets of intervention and change. Only with such vigilance can we self-consciously frame the questions that we wish to address.

There are many foundations to build upon in an effort to understand and identify social regularities. Several theories—developmental, organizational, and ecological—are particularly enlightening. Inherent in developmental theory's temporal bias is the notion of continuity and discontinuity, and its derivative concepts of stages and transitions—the latter already being fundamental to work in Community Psychology. Organizational and ecological theories are rich in relational thinking, that is, in transactional and recursive concepts. Although these theories hold great promise for the conceptual mining of social regularities, they offer few operational leads for the measurement of these phenomena.

In this chapter, I have presented some preliminary suggestions and caveats for conceptualizing and measuring social regularities. But there is considerable work to be done. Research must operationalize and measure social regularities without unwittingly slipping into the trap of attribute-centered constructs, with which we are far more comfortable and familiar. We must keep our "eyes on the prize," because it is only through the identification, measurement, and targeting of social regularities that we can begin to develop a full-blown action science of community psychology (Seidman, 1988).

CHAPTER 10

CRITERIA OF EXCELLENCE II. HYPOTHESIS GENERATION:
HUMAN SCIENCE AND ATTRIBUTE-CENTERED SOCIAL REGULARITIES

BRENNA H. BRY, BARTON J. HIRSCH, J. ROBERT NEWBROUGH,
THOMAS M. REISCHL, AND RALPH W. SWINDLE

There are at least two epistemological positions within science on the nature of knowledge to be generated. The first assumes the possibility of certain knowledge—*epistémé*, what we know to be true—and searches for the foundations for it. The other assumes the impossibility of certain foundational knowledge and pursues *apodictic* knowledge—what we believe to be true (Polkinghorne, 1983). The first is *logical positivism*, an approach developed to rid science of metaphysics and subjectivity. The second, *human science*, developed from a critical evaluation of positivism (Suppe, 1974, as quoted in Polkinghorne, 1983). Human science is based on the assumption that knowledge is limited by historical and cultural context and merely represents the best available explanation of reality (Polkinghorne, 1983).

Community psychology is of both traditions, but is conceptually more at home with the second. Community psychology developed when the experimental tradition of logical positivism was dominant. At the same time, the action-research tradition of Kurt Lewin (1951a) provided an alternative image of mission-oriented research carried out in field settings within the context of conflicting points of view. This image reflected the human science tradition, and positioned community psychology to be in pursuit of apodictic knowledge. Apodictic knowledge is generated to be both theoretically relevant and functionally useful. It is also expected that such knowledge will be superseded by improved knowledge developed through further research and action.

The inspiration for human science comes from Dilthey (1833–1911) who objected to Hobbes's description of life as a machine. Dilthey argued that life is what is experienced in activities and reflections as people live out their personal histories. Persons have to be understood in the context of their connections to cultural and social life (Polkinghorne, 1983). Both Polkinghorne (1983) and Morgan (1983) elaborated this orientation as it is expressed in methodology. The rejection of a certain epistemological foundation by the human science tradition emphasizes science as a social matter, where the researchers have to choose not only method, but conceptual positions as well. Morgan calls these latter "ontological uncertainties" that accompany the epistemological uncertainties engendered by the lack of a foundation. Citing Heisenberg's "uncertainty principle" and Bohr's "principle of complementarity," Morgan (1983) argues that "the scientist does not generate knowledge of an object world, but of his *interaction with* that world, and that science tells the scientist as much about him[self] or herself as it does about the phenomenon being investigated" (p. 387).

This interaction is called *engagement* between the scientist and the subject of study through "a particular frame of reference" (Morgan, 1983, p. 389). Morgan goes on to say that ". . . social phenomena may have many potential ways of revealing themselves, and . . . the way they are realized in practice depends on the mode of engagement adopted by the researcher" (p. 389).

The choice of perspective, method, findings (knowledge claims), and consequences is the main problem confronting the community psychology researcher. Although reliability, validity, and replicability are the traditional bases for acceptance of knowledge that is based on hypothesis-testing research, human science researchers have to engage in a social process of evaluating knowledge claims. Polkinghorne (1983) describes the use of practical reasoning and argumentation in deciding how to conduct research. Consistent with the nature of this volume, Morgan (1983) describes this process as reflective conversation among researchers, a rational approach of observing and questioning and "making intelligent choices about the means they adopt and the ends they serve" (p. 406). The goal of human science is the opposite of positivism; it is to promote improved diversity in the field. At the same time, human science looks for temporary certainty through the application of critical multiplism (Cook, 1983, 1986; Shadish, Cook, & Houts, 1986), which seeks consistency within a process of negating alternative hypotheses.

The role of the hypothesis is central to both traditions. The hypothesis reflects the scientist's belief about the way in which the phenomenon works. It serves the positivist tradition as the way to guide empirical work in the development of general laws. In the human sciences, where the metaphor of machine is

The order of the second through the fifth authors is alphabetical. Preparation of Ralph Swindle's portion of this chapter was supported by National Institute of Alcoholism and Alcohol Abuse (NIAAA) Grants AA02863 and AA06699, and by Veterans Administration Medical and Health Services Research and Development Service research funds.

not commonly held, it serves more varied functions. Among other things, it serves as a guide to location (where to look), to action (where to intervene), and to evaluation (what to consider as alternative explanations). In other words, the hypothesis is determined not only by the scientist's epistemology, but also by the scientist's worldview or conceptual context for research.

WORLDVIEW OR CONCEPTUAL CONTEXT: METAPHOR AS EXPLANATORY MODEL

Morgan (1983) suggested the use of metaphor, or explanatory model, as the primary way to communicate a scientist's conceptual context for hypothesis generation. He offered, among others, the following metaphors as applicable to social organizations: a learning system, a socially constructed reality, a life history, a theater, a system of communicative disorder, and a mode of social domination. Such metaphors may be equally applicable to the study of community and may each generate some important knowledge about it.

At present, many metaphors in community psychology research seem to deal with social inequalities. Concern was expressed at the conference at which the papers in this book were presented that the range of explanations in community psychology discourse is too circumscribed. A limited selection of metaphors is not providing enough sharp differences in the dialogue to improve thinking. This narrow range of metaphors is seen as a major problem in the field—one that requires attention and action.

SOCIAL REGULARITIES: A FOCUS FOR HYPOTHESIS GENERATION IN A HUMAN SCIENCE OF COMMUNITY PSYCHOLOGY

Seidman (see Chapter 9 in this volume) facilitates the development of a more fully articulated human science of community psychology. He concurs that the metaphors and other conceptual perspectives that provide the framework for hypothesis generation in community research are too limited. More specifically, he argues that individual attributes and linear causal models are overemphasized. Instead, he favors a focus on social regularities within and between settings. A *social regularity* is a pattern of transactions between actors over time that is connected to persons. Social regularities are constructs that enable a human science to capture the dynamic relationships between actors (persons, groups, organizations, etc.). These relationships are central to theory about the nature of community life and about the relationship of persons to their communities. More specifically, social regularities may be considered as computational relations, relational processes, and constructions of reality.

Seidman suggests two possible types of social regularities characterized as computational relations. That is, both can be represented by a mathematical relation between two units along some dimension of interest. The first type is represented by a *difference* on a substantive dimension between two units (typically social units such as groups, populations, or organizational entities). An example of such a construct would be the gender-equity orientation of an employment setting measured by the difference in salaries between men and women in the setting.

The second type is represented by a *ratio* that characterizes the relative position of a group or population to a larger organizational unit. Mulvey, Linney, and Rosenberg (1987) classified 30 residential treatment settings for juvenile offenders according to the distribution of decision-making power among staff groups and residents. The researchers identified four types of organizational control patterns:

1. *Administrative hierarchy.* Decision power was greatest among directors and decreased going down the pecking order (6 settings).
2. *Middle-level staff control.* Setting directors and residents had less power than the supervisors and line staff (11 settings).
3. *Joint staff-resident control.* Power was essentially equal among all staff groups and residents (9 settings).
4. *Equal staff control.* Staff groups had the same level of power and residents had little power (4 settings).

This social regularity (the organizational control pattern) is based on the mathematical ratios of power scores of each group to the power scores of other groups in the treatment settings.

Both the difference and ratio types of social regularities represent mathematical computations involving variables that might otherwise be considered attribute-centered constructs. Persons or groups can be characterized by the relatively stable attributes of income and power, but the same data can be used to compute difference or ratio scores that characterize social regularities at a higher level of analysis.

A second way to view social regularities is to focus directly on interactive or relational processes, rather than to compute a difference or ratio variable that reflects a relational process. For example, a directly assessed social regularity is *competitive versus cooperative learning* in classrooms. The reward systems in the competitive classroom encourage students to withhold information from other students (e.g., do homework separately). Students in cooperative learning settings, however, are encouraged to share their knowledge and experiences. The competitive–cooperative dimension could be represented by the average number of information exchanges among students in a classroom.

Third, social regularities may be thought of as constructions of reality. That is, there is a complicating, interpretive dimension to defining social regularities. Variables may be considered individual attributes or social regularities depending on the researcher's theory-in-use or nomological network for the variable. (See Chapter 10 by Seidman, in this volume.) Consider this question: Is intelligence a social regularity? In a technical sense, the intelligence quotient fits the characteristic of social regularities as mathematical relations. IQ was initially defined as a ratio of mental age divided by chronological age and more recently has been. defined relative to other IQ scores. Seidman (1988) noted that, although intelligence could be a social regularity, most researchers consider it a stable attribute of persons. Thus, in general, intelligence should be thought of as an attribute-centered construct.

Seidman also emphasized that, although social regularities may be identified at the individual level, the challenge for community researchers is to identify and to study social regularities using larger units of analysis, including the group, the organization, and the community. The earlier examples of equity orientation, organizational control pattern, and classroom interactions each characterize a group or organization. Given the importance of the researcher's theory-in-use in determining whether these variables are social regularities or individual attributes, we must also note explicitly that social regularities are theoretical abstractions of reality. For example, if the equity orientation of an organization is considered to be a static characteristic, the variable is attribute-centered. On the other hand, if the researcher's theory or organizational functioning includes axioms about the dynamic influence of income differences among men and women, then equity orientation is a social regularity.

More generally, theory-building with social regularities is fraught with opportunity. On the one hand, using such relational constructs can increase the risk of developing circular, redundant, and ambiguous theories of limited descriptive or explanatory value. On the other, social regularities can enable us to capture the complex, transactional qualities of community phenomena. They can be sensitive to change over time and to their connections to persons. They can encourage the divergent thinking needed to build a human science of community psychology.

COMMUNITY RESEARCH: CONTEXT AND TRENDS

Content analyses of articles in community psychology journals (Loo, Fong, & Iwamasa, 1988; Lounsbury, Cook, Leader, & Meares, 1985; Novaco & Monahan, 1980) and network analyses of community psychologists (Dalton, Elias, & Howe, 1985; Elias, Dalton, Franco, & Howe, 1984) yield empirical information concerning both the context of and trends within community research. These data indicate the complexities that directly and indirectly affect the relative investment of time and energy that community researchers devote to research traditions grounded in logical positivism and to those grounded in human science. In their network study of members of the American Psychological Association's Division 27, Elias et al. (1984) found that most respondents had multiple professional allegiances. First, most identified clinical or counseling psychology, not community psychology, as their major field. Second, community researchers tended to be in tenure-track positions in psychology departments and to conduct research in field settings in the community. Third, the researchers were often the sole community psychologists in their academic departments. Their colleagues evaluate them first in terms of their productivity and quality in mainstream (logical positivist tradition) terms and secondarily as community psychologists.

For junior faculty and graduate students in particular, there are, therefore, strong incentives to demonstrate expertise by publishing in a traditional area of inquiry and by using traditional methodologies, as well as by conducting innovative community research. For example, community researchers in school settings may be encouraged to address individual-level attributes of interest to developmental and clinical child psychologists and to publish in the American Psychological Association's developmental and clinical psychology journals. Thus, the research of community psychologists may be published in noncommunity journals that share the researchers' problem focus. It may become advantageous, if not necessary for researchers' academic careers, for researchers' community-based studies to generate publications and grants on traditional individual-level psychological attributes related to psychopathology, assessment, clinical intervention, and development as well as to be concerned with innovative social regularities and with new ways of examining multiple levels of analysis. Consequently, it is not surprising that, in practice, community psychologists pursue knowledge both epistemically and apodictically.

In addition to the dilemma of multiple allegiances, community psychologists face another major, if not unique, contextual problem—limited resources. Elias et al. (1984) reported that both academic and nonacademic community researchers note lack of resources for community research in their settings. Specifically, lack of funding, lack of collaborators in community research, lack of community cooperation, political obstacles such as the lack of support for nonmainstream ideologies, and lack of incentives for community research in the work setting were the major hindrances reported. (Neither lack of adequate research training nor pressure to publish, however, were nominated as problems.) Although many fields must cope with limited resources, this lack of resources can have a significant impact on fields like community psychology. Because of its youth, the field of community psychology needs to acquire resources in order to develop and to sustain emerging research relationships, settings, and traditions. Lack of resources for these developments can have a more negative impact on a younger maturing field than on a well-established one. In addition, because of their multiple allegiances, community researchers may find that limited resources may reduce their capacity to conduct adventuresome community research even further.

Given the aspirations of human science and the generation of innovative hypotheses—such as those concerning social regularities, on the one hand, and the tradition of logical positivism and the context of multiple allegiances and limited resources, on the other—what kinds of research are community psychologists publishing? Consistent with the history of logical positivism in mainstream psychology and with Seidman's critique, Lounsbury et al. (1985) reported an emphasis on individual attributes and individual levels of analysis. Thus, not enough attention has been given to systems-level constructs such as the psychological sense of community and optimal environment. In terms of multiple allegiances across respondents, Elias et al. (1984) found that one third of their respondents identified specific problem areas such as divorce, urban stress, child abuse, or alcoholism as the focus of their work in community psychology. Lounsbury and his coworkers found that fully 97 percent of the empirical research published in community journals occurs in field settings.

Interestingly, in spite of the common criticism of the constraints of the positivistic tradition, only 31 percent of the studies reviewed by Lounsbury and his colleagues (1985) stated testable hypotheses. Other articles were exploratory, descriptive, or hypothesis generating. More generally, Lounsbury and colleagues were concerned with the relative lack of theory-directed research and of generalizability of findings, with the heavy reliance on self-report measures, and with a lack of strong methodological standards. On the positive side, they noted a strong emphasis on problem-focused applied research that sought to determine the best policies and programs for a diversity of social issues. Thus, despite the potential barriers of multiple allegiances and inadequate resources, community psychology research has focused on the problems of real-world settings. Despite potent reinforcements for methodologies more consistent with logical positivism, community psychologists have shown a willingness to engage in the more exploratory, qualitative, and situation-bounded inquiries consonant with human science.

CONCLUSION: PREPARING FOR THE MOVE TO HUMAN SCIENCE

Philosophically, the context of science is changing. Community research seems poised to make a transition to placing greater emphasis on human science; community researchers are conducting studies in community settings and are seeking to solve ever-changing social problems. We are aware of the usefulness and especially of the limits of such research in the positivist tradition. Human science provides a potentially viable alternative worth exploring, and Seidman's umbrella construct of social regularities suggests a heuristically intriguing, human-science approach to generating hypotheses.

What is currently needed is a critical mass of direction, leadership, energy, and resources dedicated to pursuing excellence in community research as a human science. These will help overcome the contextual constraints of multiple allegiances and limited resources. In our view, the dialectic of constructive intellectual conflict (as well as mutual support) among researchers is essential. Through a stimulating dialectic, differences are articulated, methods for testing them are developed, research is conducted, supported elements are retained, syntheses are achieved, and new directions are indicated. In short, science progresses. In the past, among researchers, insufficient engagement and a norm of separate, independent research have slowed progress. A focused examination of different ideas, problems, and methods seems to be at the heart of human science. These will help overcome the contextual constraints of multiple allegiances and limited resources.

To promote constructive explication of differences, several possible steps would be useful. First, the discipline, like others such as biology, may choose to select a few central, high-priority research questions to emphasize for several years. Such questions could be topics for books, special issues of journals, lead articles with invited simultaneous responses, specialty conferences, and major conference addresses and symposia. Second, diverse theoretical positions such as the five in this volume (see chapters 3-7), need to be more fully developed in terms of their conceptual, methodological, and practical complexities, and complexities in underlying values, together with implications for understanding community phenomena. Underlying epistemologies need to be examined. An important complementary activity here is to become better acquainted with our conceptual roots. For example, it would be constructive to review Skinner (1953), van Bertanlaffy (1968) and Lewin (1951a,b) for what they had to say about relational phenomena, multiple levels of analysis, and recursive causal assumptions. Such an understanding of our theoretical and epistemological differences and of our heritage will provide a strong conceptual foundation for developing a human science.

Third, new research designs and methods of quantitative and qualitative analyses will be needed to capture the complexity of community phenomena. Drawing on the insights and methods of other areas of psychology and other disciplines is very useful here.

Finally, to provide a solid organizational base for the further development of community research, the creation of a variety of community research laboratories, analogous to the Woods' Hole Laboratory in marine biology and similar to the National Institute of Mental Health's Prevention Intervention Research Centers, is recommended. In such settings, focal research questions could be explored. Scholarly cross-pollination could be encouraged. The process of constructive dialectic and dialogue that was encouraged within community psychology at the Chicago conference that was the wellspring of this book should be continued and expanded to an interdisciplinary interaction.

With these opportunities for progress, community research will be able to explore the philosophical assumptions, metaphors, and overall value of the human science perspective and, in the process, build our knowledge of community phenomena. It is to be hoped that such efforts will further the development of the field as a scientific community that continually examines its criteria for knowing.

PART FOUR

LEVELS OF ANALYSIS: LOOKING AT THE PERSON AND THE SETTING

CHAPTER 11

MIXING AND MATCHING:
LEVELS OF CONCEPTUALIZATION, MEASUREMENT, AND STATISTICAL ANALYSIS IN COMMUNITY RESEARCH

MARYBETH SHINN

Levels of analysis that go beyond the individual to incorporate ever-broader contexts of behavior are central to community psychology. Members of the field (Murrell, 1973; Rappaport, 1977; Seidman, 1988) and fellow travellers (Altman & Rogoff, 1987; Bronfenbrenner, 1979, 1986) have proposed schemata for levels of analysis in order to clarify the concept and to exhort community psychologists to include "higher" levels in theory and research. Higher levels may be distinguished from lower ones in three respects: They may involve (a) multiple individuals, for example, populations (Murrell, 1973; Seidman, 1988); (b) units with internal structure and social organization, for example, groups or organizations (Rappaport, 1977); and (c) patterns of interactions or reciprocal relations between individuals, groups, and social systems, for example, settings (Seidman, 1988), the organismic worldview (Altman & Rogoff, 1987), mesosystems (Bronfenbrenner, 1979, 1986; Seidman, 1988), and intersystem or network interventions (Murrell, 1973). In the extreme, represented by the worldview that Altman and Rogoff (1987) call *transactional*, the entities disappear into "a *confluence* of inseparable factors that depend on one another for their very definition and meaning" (p. 24), and relationships become paramount. Several of these definitions of levels implicitly consider the physical or social environment of behavior, and in my discussion, I will include the environment as an extraindividual unit of analysis.

Community research frequently deals with populations, ignoring social structure, as in many studies of prevention, and with patterns of relations among individuals, as in studies of social networks. It has been less successful, however, in understanding social structures and patterns of reciprocal relations that involve units at higher levels. I attribute this lack of success both to conceptual problems in understanding the role of variables at different levels of analysis and to methodological problems in selecting strategies for measurement and statistical analysis that are suitable for research that goes beyond the individual.

I will begin by discussing conceptual issues regarding higher levels of analysis. Next, I will describe problems and partial solutions to the problem of measuring extraindividual phenomena using information about individuals that focuses on issues of subjectivity and aggregation. In brief interlude, I ponder why psychologists typically attempt to assess higher-level phenomena by "asking individuals." The final section considers measures of extraindividual units that match the level of conceptualization.

CONCEPTUAL PROBLEMS

Cross-Level and Multilevel Research

Rousseau (1985) developed a typology of research involving multiple levels in organizations. Her concept of *level* embodies the first two of the characteristics that I listed as distinguishing between levels and adds the notion of a hierarchical relationship between levels. For Rousseau, higher levels are larger and more complex than lower ones, but they are essentially *entities* characterized by distinctive structures and processes, rather than *patterns* of mutual influence, or, in Seidman's terms (see Chapter 9 in this volume), *attribute-centered constructs* rather than *social regularities*. Relationships are the focus of cross-level and multilevel research.

Rousseau (1985, p. 16) identified three types of *cross-level* relationships (also called *mixed-level*; e.g., Glick, 1980); (a) a relationship among variables at different levels, such as the relationship between school environment and children's attendance or achievement (e.g., Felner, Ginter, & Primavera, 1982); (b) a moderating effect of a variable from one level on a relationship between variables at another, such as a difference in the relationship between perceived stressors and experienced distress in more and less supportive settings (e.g., Maton, 1989); and (c) the effect of individual differences from a group standard or a "frog-pond effect" (Firebaugh, 1980), such as relative, rather than absolute, poverty (e.g., Seidman & Rapkin, 1983).

I thank the organizers, of the September 1988 conference on which this volume is based—Fern Chertok, Leonard Jason, Christopher Keys, and, especially, Patrick Tolan—and respondents LaRue Allen, Cary Cherniss, Bill Davidson, Maurice Elias, and Allan Wicker for their thoughtful comments on an earlier version of this chapter. My New York University colleagues Barbara Felton, Diane Hughes, Bruce Rapkin, and Edward Seidman pushed me to clarify my thoughts and to follow out their implications with comments at once trenchant and gentle. Fred Dansereau, Rosalie Hall, Dennis Perkins, and Abraham Wandersman kindly sent me materials on the Butterfly Consortium, which Abe organized to think about statistical issues in levels of analysis. Kenneth Maton, Ralph Swindle, and Alan Wicker introduced me to other valuable materials.

Multilevel research concerns relationships between independent and dependent variables at a given level that replicate across two or more levels. In an example also cited by Rousseau (1985), Staw, Sandelands, and Dutton (1981) reviewed evidence indicating that individuals, groups, and organizations respond similarly to threat, that is, an environmental event with impending negative or harmful consequences for the entity. At each level, threat leads to restriction in information and constriction in control and, consequently, to well-learned, dominant, or rigid responses. Staw et al. (1981) hypothesized that such responses are adaptive when environmental changes are small but that they are potentially maladaptive under conditions of great turbulence or radical change.

Multilevel research may have considerable power to generate hypotheses about the applicability of understanding garnered at one level to constructs and processes at another level. For example, hypotheses about the differential effectiveness of problem-focused and emotion-focused coping at the individual level might be extended to group-level coping activities, under the rubric of *social support*, and to activities undertaken by organizations to assist members (Shinn, Morich, Robinson, & Neuner, 1986). But multilevel theories are as likely to obscure as to clarify if they are only anthropomorphic metaphors (e.g., Rousseau, 1985). To exploit multilevel models requires a *composition theory* that specifies the relationships between variables at different levels presumed to be functionally similar (Roberts, Hulin, & Rousseau, 1978, p. 84; Rousseau, 1985). The notion of environmental threat, for example, is more similar across individuals, groups, and organizations than is the notion of constriction of control. Content theories, describing relationships among variables, and process theories, describing how constructs are combined to produce responses (Roberts et al., 1978, p. 84), may also vary across levels.

I contend that most research in community psychology is, or ought to be, cross-level in nature. This goal is reflected in the oxymoronic nature of the field's name. *Community* refers to extraindividual (group, organizational, setting, mesosystem) contexts; *psychology* refers to individual experience (cf. Keys & Frank, 1987a). Constructs such as *empowerment* or *person–environment fit* are exciting when they embody a cross-level relationship between the individual and the social system. When they are defined in terms of individual psychological variables, say *locus of control* for empowerment or *satisfaction with the environment* for person–environment fit, they lose their community flavor. Although community psychologists may be concerned with relationships between settings or with effective functioning of groups or organizations as targets of research or intervention, we study these higher levels of analysis not just for their own sake but for their impact on individual well-being. Were we to lose this ultimate connection to the individual, we would cease to be psychologists; but when we confine ourselves to the individual level, we lose our community identity.

Cross-level models typically involve a downward flow of influence from higher to lower levels of analysis, but this downwardness is not inherent in the concept (Rousseau, 1985). Community psychologists who study social change, for example, invoke cross-level models in which individuals or groups influence larger social units or create new settings. Bidirectional models are also possible.

Mismatch Between Level of Conceptualization and Level of Measurement

So far I have used the term *level* to mean what Katz and Kahn (1978, p. 13) called "level of conceptualization" and Rousseau (1985) called "focal unit," that is, the level of theory or understanding—the level at which conclusions are drawn and generalizations are made. In practice, the level of conceptualization may differ from the level at which data are collected—the level of measurement (Rousseau, 1985) or level of phenomenon (Katz & Kahn, 1978)—and the level to which data are assigned for statistical analysis (Rousseau, 1985). A central question for community research concerns the consequences of a mismatch between level of conceptualization and level of measurement.

Lewin (1946/1952) argued that, whereas it is possible objectively and reliably to measure units of any size with methods fitted to the unit, the "attempt to determine reliably large macroscopic units by observing microscopic units...is bound to fail" (p. 244). Katz and Kahn, on the other hand, held that researchers must distinguish between levels of conceptualization and levels of measurement, but that the two need not match. Although levels of conceptualization and measurement covary in the natural sciences, so that, for example, the psychological experiences of color vision cannot be fully understood by measuring the physiological processes, in the social sciences, higher-level (emergent) phenomena may be observed in the interrelated actions of individuals. Katz and Kahn continue:

> Our thesis, then, is that the study of organizations should take the social system level as its conceptual starting point, but that many of the actual measures will be constructed from observations and reports of individual behavior and attitude. Concepts at the system level tell us what particular individual data to gather and how to use them. In studying the introduction of a new piece rate into an industrial enterprise, an individually-oriented psychologist might concentrate on the worker's needs for economic gains. The system-oriented social psychologist would look for the group norms that legitimate production rates. Both researchers would have to observe the behavior of individuals and both would have to put their questions to individuals, but their foci of inquiry and their inferences from data would be different.[1]

The assertion that one can assess extraindividual units of conceptualization by questioning individuals requires scrutiny. Consider the examples of economic needs and group norms in more detail. It is not hard to imagine ways of assessing workers' needs for economic gains by questioning individuals. If need is defined by an individual's subjective state, there may be no better approach. But norms

---

[1]From *The Social Psychology of Organizations* (2nd ed., p. 13) by D. Katz and R. L. Kahn. Copyright 1978, New York, John Wiley & Sons. Reprinted by permission.

are considered not simply as cognitive expectations but as social standards that regulate attitude and behavior (e.g., Sherif, 1936, p. 85), it is less clear that individual perceptions are a good way to measure them. Should the researcher ask individuals directly about the existence or strength of norms or the extent to which they are shared and, then, *average* the responses? Or should he or she ask each individual what the presumed norms are and then look at the *variability* of responses? Does disagreement indicate lack of norms, lack of reliability in measuring them, or perhaps the existence of subgroups for whom norms operate in very different ways? To answer these questions, we need more insight into both problems in measuring extraindividual phenomena by collecting data from individuals and (as Katz and Kahn, 1978, put it) into how data from individuals should be used to shed light on higher levels of conceptualization.

MEASURING EXTRAINDIVIDUAL PHENOMENA USING INFORMATION FROM INDIVIDUALS

Problems of Subjectivity

One set of problems in measuring extraindividual phenomena by questioning individuals involves subjectivity: Different people describe the phenomenon differently. Before consigning such differences to error variance, it is important to consider their causes. First, people encounter distinct subenvironments in systematic and random ways. Opportunities, for example, vary systematically for individuals by race, sex, class, or place in an organization's structure. (The tourist whose pocket happens to get picked has a lower impression of the city than one whose experiences are more benign.) Second, perception is inherently an act of interpretation, and people bring assorted frames of reference to phenomena. Individual differences may be systematic and stable due, for example, to history, culture, or cognitive style; they may change predictably owing to psychological development or to changing needs or experience in a setting; or they may be asystematic (cf. James & Sells, 1981; Jessor & Jessor, 1973).

Golembiewski, Billingsley, and Yeager (1976), showed how systematic modifications in perspective can create difficulties in measuring social change. They assessed individuals' perceptions of the authority structure of their organization before and after an intervention that was designed to increase levels of participation in decision making. Although respondents agreed at posttest that the environment was more participatory than before, direct comparison of pre- and posttest scores indicated a shift in the opposite direction. Golembiewski et al. (1976) suggested that the intervention did change the organization in the direction of greater participation but that it changed the respondents' vision of participatory processes even more, so that the discrepancy between vision and reality increased. One may attempt to eliminate such stretching of perceptual yardsticks by anchoring rating scales, or one may study it as a phenomenon of interest, but one ignores it at one's peril.

If individual perceptions of extraindividual phenomena are joint functions of person and phenomenon, it is not surprising that efforts to measure person and environment variables separately by means of individual perceptions and to compare the two as a measure of person–environment fit (e.g., French, Rodgers, & Cobb, 1974) have been less fruitful than once hoped. A similar problem arises for measures of discrepancy between real and ideal social climates. Part of the variance in the conceptual variable of fit or discrepancy is already captured in individual perceptions of the "real" environment. For example, a person judging the truth of items such as "This is a lively place" or "Members are pretty busy all of the time" (Community Oriented Programs Environment Scale; Moos, 1974) would probably compare the degree of liveliness or busyness to internal standards. In fact, individual ratings of the environment might themselves be conceptualized as measures of person–environment fit.

Partial Solutions to Problems of Subjectivity

Different frames of reference do not make individual reports of extraindividual phenomena worthless. As Lewin (1943a) pointed out, community life would be impossible if our social observations were not reasonably accurate. Individual differences in perception may be reduced or modeled, depending on their causes.

To reduce error variance from asystematic differences in frames of reference or from systematic differences that one is willing to treat as unwanted bias, one can make questions more objective. Standard techniques include anchoring rating scales, using comparison objects or vignettes to create common frames of reference, or asking about specific behaviors or objective facts rather than about inherently subjective phenomena. Wherever possible, the construct validity of such quasi-objective self-report measures should be assessed rather than assumed.

In the pursuit of quasi-objective self-reports, one should be wary of pseudo-objectivity. High correlations between measures that are designed to be either purely descriptive or purely affective confirm the importance of attitude to perception (Guion, 1973). Counts of subjectively defined entities (e.g., the number of people in a social network) are unlikely to be more objective than ratings of more frankly subjective events (e.g., perceived social support).

Because individual differences in perspective may feed into both independent and dependent measures (whether within or between levels), inflating relationships between them, relationships are more credible when both measures are not contaminated by viewing them through the same perceptual lens. For example, Repetti (1987) showed that workers' perceptions of their job environment were related to their coworkers' psychological outcomes. Billings and Moos (1982) found that wives' perceptions of stress in their own work environments were associated with their husbands' self-reports of symptoms. Of course, members of an interacting group or family, as in the examples above, may share a common frame of reference, so that "contamination" is not eliminated. Thus, Maton's (1989) finding that group-level social support and cohesion, as judged by aggregates of individual perceptions, were related to individual outcomes, even after controlling for effects of the individual's own perceptions of support, is especially impressive.

Another approach to reduce all types of bias is to use independent, trained observers to assess environments or phenomena at extraindividual levels of analysis. Murray (1938), for example, defined *environmental press* as the effects that the situation "is exerting or could exert upon the organism" (p. 40), but to avoid circularity in inferring the stimulus from the response, he distinguished between *alpha press* "that actually exists, as far as scientific inquiry can determine it" and *beta press*, which is filtered through the individual's perceptions (p. 122). Although he assessed only beta press, he suggested measuring alpha press by means of the "judgments of disinterested trained observers" (p. 290). Chein (1954) similarly advocated a middle ground between the Gestalt psychologists' geographical (objective, physical) and behavioral (perceived, social) environments. He proposed a geobehavioral or objective–behavioral environment—that is, the environment looked at objectively from the point of view of understanding behavior.

An important advance in Chein's thinking, from the perspective of today's community psychology, is his prescient understanding that a single geographical environment may correspond to different objective–behavioral environments for different groups, for example, men and women or Blacks and Whites. These differences, he contended, can be understood without abandoning the geobehavioral environment for a psychological analysis of individuals.[2]

The literature on predicting psychological dysfunction from stressful life events illustrates these different approaches. A central issue concerns who should rate the stressfulness of (or degree of change caused by) events. Sarason, Johnson, and Siegel (1978) held that respondents themselves are in the best position to rate the events that they experience, a stance that has been criticized as confounding ratings of stressfulness with the distress that the events produce. Dohrenwend, Krasnoff, Askenasy, and Dohrenwend (1978) used samples of raters that were matched with respondents on demographic characteristics. The matching allowed them to model the different cultural meanings that diverse groups attach to events. Even so, their approach has been criticized as losing unique features of the objective situation. Brown and Harris (1978) assessed the stressfulness of given events in the context of respondents' lives. Their "contextual" ratings "were designed to record what most women would have felt given the particular circumstances—past and present—of the individual woman" who experienced the event (p. 274). The method is highly idiographic, but attempts to assess the objective–behavioral environment separately from the individual's personality or responses.

---

[2]Ideas, such as *behavior*, can be understood better in context. Chein worked on the social scientists' brief for *Brown v. Board of Education* (1954: 347 U.S. 483) at about the time he wrote his article; whereas Murray, 16 years earlier, developed his theory in a study of 50 White male Harvard students.

Assessment by key informants is a technique representing a middle ground between assessment by members of an interacting group and assessment by independent observers. Key informants typically have better access to the phenomena on which they are asked to report than do observers from a research team, but they are typically neither so well-trained to common yardsticks for measurement nor so independent. In using key informants, it is important to assess their orientations and take them into account. Otherwise, the technique will not eliminate problems of subjectivity, but simply hide them (James, Joyce, & Slocum, 1988, p. 131).

Both observers and key informants, at their best, may provide insight not only into the extraindividual phenomenon, but also into systematic differences in the perceptions of others and the reasons for them. They offer a level of theoretical abstraction and interpretation unavailable to the participant *qua* participant (Stern, 1970, p. 7).

The standard wisdom is that triangulation of multiple sources of measurement will bring the researcher closer to "truth" (e.g., Campbell & Fiske, 1959; Webb, Campbell, Schwartz, Sechrest, & Grove, 1981). My position is a variant: Multiple sources yield multiple truths. The researcher's job is to understand and to model the individual and extraindividual sources of variance.

Problems of Aggregation

Another approach to characterizing extraindividual units is to aggregate information from the individuals who make them up. Either individual perceptions of the unit (as in the case of social climate) or other demographic, social, or behavioral characteristics of the individuals within the unit (Moos, 1973) may be aggregated. This approach assumes that individual biases cancel out, yielding a more reliable and valid picture of the whole. The validity of the assumption depends on the sources of individual variance.

Both the advantages and difficulties of aggregation are illustrated in the literature about social and organizational climates. Theorists debate whether *climate* is properly a psychological or an environmental variable (see Hall, 1988, for an excellent review).

James (1982; James & Sells, 1981; James et al., 1988) held that climate is an individual variable. Psychological climates are cognitive representations of environments "in terms of their psychological meaning and significance to the individual" (James, 1982, p. 219). To the extent that individuals agree, climate perceptions may be aggregated to describe "how individuals in general impute meaning to environments" (1982, p. 220), and this aggregate or organizational climate has the same status for groups, in a composition theory, as perceived climate at the individual level. In this view, organizational climate is simply the central tendency of individual perceptions. The unit of theory is still the individual (James, 1982; James et al., 1988). In an example that shows just how ready proponents of this orientation are to dispense with organizations in assessing climate, Joyce and Slocum (1984) cluster analyzed climate scores to form artificial groups of people whose perceived "organizational" climates were similar but who did not share a common place in the organizational structure.

For Glick (1985, 1988), on the other hand, the idea that the existence of organizational climate depends on interrater agreement is intolerable. Following Geertz (1973), he contended that shared meanings are social and public, not individual phenomena. Organizational climate is an irreducible emergent property of the organization and not simply an aggregate of psychological processes. Similarly, Moos held that climate or the "personality" of the setting describes environmental dimensions "with a great deal of accuracy and detail" (Moos, 1976, p. 320), although more recently he viewed "perceptions of social climate" as emerging from an interplay between the "actual" environment and individual values and beliefs (Moos, 1986, p. 14).

The disparate views of climate have led to different strategies for measurement and criteria for aggregation. Glick (1985) held that, if climate is an organizational variable, one should assess it in multiple ways, including (but not limited to) individual perceptions. Similarly, Moos and Lemke (e.g., 1984) have measured program environments in multiple ways (without claiming that all reflect social climate). The focus of perceptual questions also differs. That is, whereas James et al. (1988) proposed asking individuals about their own experiences, Glick (1985) proposed asking them about the organization; and whereas James et al. (1988) allowed for units of climate between the individual and the organization on the basis of degree of agreement at each level, Glick (1985) required that the level be built into the assessment instrument.

Guion (1973) suggested that perceptions be accepted as measures of organizational attributes only if they are virtually unanimous. James (1982) also placed great weight on measures of interrater agreement. Glick (1985) eschewed agreement among individuals as a criterion for reliability of an organizational attribute and instead emphasized the extent to which organizations can be reliably differentiated from one another. Joyce and Slocum (1984) adopted both these criteria for construct validity and added a third: predictable relationships between climate and other variables at organizational or individual levels.

Social climates that are based on aggregated perceptions within intact groups have had impressive successes along Joyce and Slocum's third criterion of predicting other group or organizational phenomena. To cite just two examples of criteria that share no perceptual method bias with climate: Classroom climates that are task-oriented and set specific academic goals while maintaining both supportive relations and structure are associated with gains on standardized achievement tests; treatment climates that lack peer or staff support, are disorganized, and have unclear rules and procedures have high dropout rates (Moos, 1984).

So far, I have described problems in assigning aggregate perceptual measures of extraindividual units to individual or extraindividual levels of analysis. Perceptual measures share another problem with other sorts of aggregate measures: Disparate relationships may be found in analyses at different levels of aggregation, and attempts to generalize from one level to another can yield serious errors in inference. Sociologists have dubbed such errors *ecological fallacies*, ever since Robinson (1950) first demonstrated the problem, but community psychologists may be more familiar with the terms *fallacy of the wrong level* or *error of logical types* (Rappaport, 1977, p. 135; Watzlawick, Weakland, & Fisch, 1974, p. 6). For example, the determinants of homelessness are probably quite different at the levels of cities and of individuals. At the city level, rates of homelessness are probably well determined by the low-income housing ratio, that is the ratio between the number of households who can afford only low-income housing to the number of low-income units available (McChesney, 1988). Predictors at the individual level include individual characteristics and circumstances. From the perspective of a city-level analysis, studies of individuals are studies in vulnerability. In McChesney's (1988) analogy, homelessness is like a game of musical chairs: the low-income housing ratio determines the number of chairs; individual factors determine only who will be left standing when the music stops.

Effects in aggregated data are effects of central tendencies or, in Firebaugh's (1980) terminology, *contextual effects*. *Deviations* from the central tendency, or *frog-pond effects* (Firebaugh, 1980), may also affect individual outcomes. Individual differences from an aggregate may imply diversity and pluralism, or they may indicate poor person–environment fit. Wechsler and Pugh (1967) showed that rates of first admissions to mental hospitals in Massachusetts among people with specific demographic characteristics (age, marital status, birthplace, profession) were higher in communities where those characteristics were relatively rare than in communities where they were common. Brown (1968) showed that college students randomly assigned to live on floors of a residence hall where few others shared their academic interests were more likely to change their majors and became less certain of their career goals than students in the majority, regardless of initial interests. Moos (1976) and Seidman and Rapkin (1983) cite other examples of frog-pond effects. Sometimes, as in the examples above, discrepancies from group norms in either direction may put individuals at risk. In other cases, only deficits, such as relative poverty, are problematic.

Statistical Solutions to Problems of Aggregation and Their Limitations

Statistical techniques can help determine whether aggregate data can be interpreted as reflecting group-level phenomena, individual-level phenomena, or both (Dansereau, Alutto, Markham, & Dumas, 1982; Dansereau, Alutto, & Yammarino, 1984; Dansereau & Markham, 1987; Glick & Roberts, 1984; Kenny, 1985; Kenny & La Voie, 1985; see also Hall, 1988, for a review, and Florin, Giamartino, Kenny & Wandersman, 1988, for an example in community research). The specifics of such analyses are beyond the scope of this chapter. Dansereau et al. (1982, 1984; Dansereau & Markham, 1987) provide a comprehensive heuristic for describing relationships among variables and entities (levels). Their methods test whether a group-level effect is best understood as working within or between groups and allow for multiple variables and conditional relationships. Kenny's (1985) "generalized group effect model" estimates each level of effect controlling for the other and provides for quantitative analysis of frog-pond effects and other group-level phenomena such as group polarization and transmission of group culture across "generations." These approaches open up exciting possibilities for exploring extraindividual levels of analysis in community research, but they are not a panacea. Both issues of methodology and of interpretation remain.

First, groups and organizations frequently have fuzzy boundaries, making it difficult to determine who is part of a group. Such fuzziness may be especially common in voluntary associations. For example, between a quarter and a third of dues-paying members of self-help groups in two studies (Hinrichsen, Revenson, & Shinn, 1985; Videka, 1979) had never attended a meeting of the club or had not done so in the past year. Cluster analysis, as proposed by Joyce and Slocum (1984), may help to determine group membership by indicating which of the available objective indicators of structure have psychological meaning. But cluster analysis without reference to structural characteristics classifies individual perceptions, rather than delineating group membership. Sociometric methods may also be used to define groups who share interpersonal environments (Schneider & Reichers, 1983).

Second, as I have noted, a given environment may provide disparate subenvironments for subgroups of individuals. A community psychology that values cultural relativity must recognize that groups often view extraindividual phenomena through distinctive lenses; settings that foster the growth of one group may do so at the expense of another. If groups are already defined, the statistical techniques may be used to apportion variance between groups and individuals or to distinguish within-group from between-group effects. If groups are not recognized, however, systematic variance that could be linked to them is lumped with individual variance. Again, sociometric or cluster analyses, with reference to what we know about achieved and ascribed status, social or organizational structure, or penetration into behavior settings (Barker, 1968, p. 51) may define meaningful subgroups.

A final statistical limitation to efforts to untangle group and individual phenomena is the fact that sample sizes at the group level are often small. A study of a complex intervention designed to change an organization with thousands of members is essentially a case study at the organizational level, and studies of more than a handful of groups or organizations are rare. Thus, quantitative techniques for assessing differences across organizations, whether by aggregation of individual responses or by direct measurement of organizational characteristics, will typically be fairly crude. Qualitative and historical techniques may be richer sources of understanding. The bias of our discipline toward quantification should not blind us to other ways of knowing (see Chapter 5, by Riger, in this volume). Of course, qualitative researchers are not immune to the errors of level described here.

Even if a researcher has identified an appropriate extraindividual unit of analysis, problems of interpretation remain. In the case of group agreement as to social climate, for example, it is important to understand the etiology of the climate, or the causes of shared perceptions. Schneider and Reichers (1983) describe three mechanisms: common experiences of the objective environment, social interaction leading to a shared social construction of reality, and grouping of individuals who share common perspectives via selection, attraction, and attrition. Settings select and reject or eject members, just as members choose settings (Barker, 1968, p. 171; Wicker, 1972). Thus, agreement among members in describing a group or organization, although an extraindividual phenomenon, may reflect more than just the objective environment. Distinguishing among sources of agreement is critical to developing interventions to promote change. Similarly, in evaluating voluntary "treatments," such as membership in self-help groups, one must distinguish group-level effects that reflect what goes on in the group from effects arising from selection, attraction, and attrition of group members. The techniques for apportioning variance are not sufficient here.

Finally, statistical solutions do not solve conceptual problems of choosing the right level at which to ask questions. Explaining variance at one level does not mean that causality operates at that level alone.

INTERLUDE: WHY ARE WE WEDDED TO MEASURING EXTRAINDIVIDUAL PHENOMENA BY QUESTIONING INDIVIDUALS?

Before turning to examples in which measurement matches the level of conceptualization, it is useful to consider why psychologists have been so wedded to measurement at the level of individual reports. I count at least two reasons: confusion between the consciously perceived environment and the functionally significant environment, and relative poverty of psychological theory at extraindividual levels.

The first confusion is illustrated in (although hardly unique to) a generally insightful article by Jessor and Jessor (1973). The authors distinguished between distal environments that are relatively "remote from direct experience" and "for the most part without immediate functional significance for the actor" and proximal "environments of perception, experience, or functional stimulation"—environments of interpretation or meaning (p. 805). The two-pronged definitions implicitly incorporate a theory that only what is consciously experienced has direct implications for behavior (cf. James & Sells, 1981).

There are studies that seem to support the notion that the perceived environment is more closely related to behavior than is the objective environment. For example, organizational structure is generally less related to behavior than is organizational climate (e.g., Lawler, Hall, & Oldham, 1974), and Moos (1986) suggested that the latter mediates the former.

Despite the weight of tradition, I believe, with Chein (1954), that it is important to divorce the notion of functional significance from that of awareness. Jessor and Jessor (1973) demonstrated that not all aspects of the perceived environment are equally influential. Moreover, both aspects of the physical environment (Proshansky, Ittelson, & Rivlin, 1970) and cultural belief systems (Maruyama, 1983, Sherif, 1936) can exert powerful influences on behavior without entering conscious awareness. Awareness is most likely when environmental forces run counter to personal needs (Barker, 1987b). In fact, one technique for reducing the pervasive influence of cultural norms is to heighten awareness of them, as in consciousness-raising in regard to norms governing male and female sex role behavior in our own culture.

Although conscious awareness is a faulty guide to functional significance, confusion would not have arisen were it not often a useful guide. Alternatives to individual reports in assessing extraindividual units too frequently ignore functional significance. This is the problem of poverty of theory noted earlier. For example, it is not surprising that measures of organizational structure, such as size, number of levels in the hierarchy, or span of control, bear scant relationship to behavior, because relevance to behavior was not a criterion in choosing them. Similarly, Rousseau (1985) complained that setting-level moderators of individual-level relations are often invoked atheoretically when a relationship holds in some settings but not in others. Poverty of theory may explain McGrath and Altman's (1966, p. 35) observation (cited by Wicker in Chapter 12A in this volume) that significant relationships between entities at different levels are rare in small-group research. The greater likelihood of significance when the same source (e.g., an individual) rates both entities may simply cast doubt on whether the entities as assessed are in fact at different levels (i.e., doubt as to the construct validity of the measures).

MEASURES THAT MATCH THE LEVEL OF CONCEPTUALIZATION

Issues in Developing Measures

Focusing on the distinction between conscious awareness and functional significance may help us to abandon the first in favor of the second as a criterion for developing measures at extraindividual units of analysis. A first step is to use theory to guide us to constructs of potential functional significance. Seidman's (1988) notion of social regularities may be especially fertile ground for cultivating such theory. For example, it was the genius of Barker and colleagues (Barker & Gump, 1974; Wicker, McGrath, & Armstrong, 1972) to translate the distal variable of organizational size into the more proximal social regularity of manning or staffing, or the relationship of the number of setting inhabitants to the number of social roles available. With the conceptualization phrased in terms of social regularities rather than physical entities, it was easier to see differences in tolerance for diversity and in mechanisms for regulating behavior in under- and overstaffed settings. In the case of type of setting as a moderator variable, the theoretical challenge is to find the social regularities that differentiate settings. Doing so will advance our understanding of the contexts of individual (or group or organizational behavior) and clarify the ecological validity of our theories. At this stage, functional significance rather than objectivity is of key importance. As Lewin (1943a) warned, the pursuit of objectivity may lead researchers to turn to measures of phenomena that are too small or too removed from context or from an interpretive framework to be useful.

A second step is to establish the construct validity of measures. Cronbach and Meehl's (1955) recommendations to elaborate the nomological network in which the construct is embedded and to specify places where the network makes contact with observations remain essential. Extending the notion of construct validity to extraindividual units of analysis additionally requires a theory of composition to specify the relationship between similar constructs at different levels (Roberts et al., 1978; Rousseau, 1985). Measures that do not match the level of conceptualization require special evidence of construct validity.

An Extended Example

Consider the example of group-level measures of norms that legitimate production rates in a piecework system. One measure would be the distribution of production rates within the group. Piecework norms imply a ceiling on individual production, with negative sanctions for rate busters. If all group members were equally capable and motivated to achieve, then all would perform at or near the ceiling, and the overall distribution would be narrow. If not all workers were sufficiently motivated or capable of attaining the norm, the distribution would be skewed, with a long tail at lower rates of production, a mode at the norm, and an immediate drop to or near zero frequency above the norm. In self-report measures, those whose production was far below the norm might not be aware of its existence; those performing at or near the norm, especially those with strong economic needs to go beyond it, might be acutely aware. Hence, lack of agreement on norms might reflect differential places in the distribution rather than lack of norms. Cross-time data would allow additional measures. If a production ceiling were the result of natural limits on skill or technology, workers' learning curves might approach it with gradual deceleration and would never exceed the limit (of course, this would be subject to minor fluctuations). If the ceiling were the result of social norms, the deceleration might be abrupt, and individuals might exceed the ceiling before being brought back into line.

Distributions of learning achievements and production rates are, of course, aggregates of individual phenomena, but with a difference. If the production rates are seen as individual measures, each individual datum has the same status as any other. The mean of production rates is simply an average of individual-level measures. If production rates are seen as part of a distribution, however, then each has meaning only as it relates to the overall pattern. The social regularity embodied in that pattern is a group-level indicator of the norm under investigation (cf. McGrath & Altman, 1966, p. 19).

Other measures of group norms might involve their transmission during the socialization process for new group members or the pressures (which Barker, 1968, called *deviation-countering circuits*), that are brought to bear on rate busters. Both the distribution of production and the particular group members subject to pressure would differ greatly under a system in which members were rewarded for the *group's* performance. In a piecework system, sanctions would be reserved for those whose production was too great; in a group-reward system, sanctions, or assistance, would be offered to those whose production was too low. Newcomers might be ignored in the first system until they became a threat; in the second, they might be singled out for help to bring them up to par. Thus, the larger social context, in this case the reward structure, should be considered in evaluating group norms.

Selected Empirical Examples
A switch to a new paradigm, as Kuhn (1970) showed, requires not only dissatisfaction with the old, but also a relatively successful, or at least promising, alternative. Thus, it is important to offer empirical examples of successful efforts to match level of measurement to level of conceptualization. The special issue of the *American Journal of Community Psychology* on organizational perspectives edited by Keys and Frank (1987b) presents a remarkable compendium; because of space constraints, I will mention only two examples.

The Blakely et al. (1987) study of dissemination of innovative social programs provides setting-level measures of the fidelity of replications to original model programs. (This study, which examined 10 efforts to replicate each of 7 programs, for 70 replications in all, is a striking exception to the rule that studies of organizations have small sample sizes.) Blakely et al. took an idiographic approach to each of the 7 original programs, identifying, with the help of program staff, ideal, acceptable, and unacceptable variations of 60 to 100 program features for each model. They also selected appropriate criteria for effectiveness (individual-level outcomes) for each model. They then visited each replication, rated its fidelity to the previously identified program features, and classified all innovative features as additions, adaptations, or unacceptable variants of the model. The cross-level conclusion—that effectiveness of replications was positively associated with fidelity of programs to the original model and to local additions but was unrelated to adaptations—has considerable ecological validity.

Gruber and Trickett (1987) used a qualitative and historical analysis over 14 years to study efforts to empower parents and students in an alternative public school. Although equal numbers of teachers, parents, and students were represented on the school's policy council, teachers grew over time, to dominate the group. The authors suggested that the teachers' greater power in the council was based on their roles in the school, responsibility for the council, knowledge of the immediate school situation, educational expertise, and control over implementation of council decisions. A central question in the article is whether it is possible to empower others. Gruber and Trickett's (1987) conclusion is not that empowerment, like dieting or jogging, is something one must do for oneself. Rather, they suggest that greater structuring of the board's leadership, agenda, and domain might have defined roles for students and parents and counterbalanced teacher's power. Paradoxically, it was the school's egalitarian ideology that stood in the way of such structuring and, hence, of empowerment. The insight into the process of empowerment garnered from careful analysis over time in this single case study should convince the most hardened data-analyst of the value of qualitative and historical work at the organizational level.

CONCLUSION

In sum, community psychology needs to pay more than lip service to issues of level in developing theory, defining variables, and testing relationships. Mixing and matching levels of conceptualization, measurement, and statistical analysis can lead to serious errors of inference. There are promising statistical techniques for extracting information about extraindividual units and relationships from data collected about or from individuals, but these techniques are not without limitations. They can aid but not substitute for clearer thinking about issues of level. With better conceptualization, we can also develop more measures that match the level of theory.

CHAPTER 12

THEORETICAL PERSPECTIVES AND LEVELS OF ANALYSIS

A. LEVELS OF ANALYSIS AS AN ECOLOGICAL ISSUE IN THE RELATIONAL PSYCHOLOGIES

ALLAN W. WICKER

How to deal with the linkage between individuals and larger social units is or should be a key conceptual concern for all of the "relational psychologies": community, social, school, organizational, and environmental. Each of these psychological specialties considers the person, or individual system, in relation to a surrounding social or sociophysical unit.

In the preceding chapter Shinn brings into focus several important aspects of the levels-of-analysis issue—most notably its conceptualization—and some methodological tactics for incorporating both individual- and community-level variables.

The following comments consider briefly these and several other facets of the issue.

STATING THE PROBLEM

Many discussions of this topic implicitly use a stair-step metaphor that is applied to two levels of analysis—the person and a larger social unit that influences that person. To help expand our perspective on the problem, I prefer the imagery of a stream, with a continual flow of events over time. Within the flow are the particular events that we focus on for study. We can situate these events in nested hierarchical systems that have temporal, spatial/physical, and relational dimensions.

A researcher who is interested in unemployment, for example, might initially focus on the personal experiences and coping strategies of the unemployed. Although unemployed individuals could be studied simply in terms of their perspectives and their actions, the ecological perspective that most of us subscribe to, coupled with perspective gained from the stream metaphor, would dictate a more complex analysis—one that is both hierarchical and dynamic. They would show the need to situate the unemployed in particular behavior settings, social groupings, and institutions. And we would then consider the temporal patterns of both the focal events and their contexts.

Although individual-level analyses in field settings are themselves often difficult to conceptualize and to carry out, embracing the stream metaphor further complicates our task by directing attention to the dynamics of cross-level transactions. We would need to consider, for example, how changes in individuals' feelings and coping strategies affect and are affected by family interactions. We should also consider how concrete enactments of economic assistance programs affect target individuals and their families, and how individual and family actions shape those enactments.

THE EPISTEMOLOGICAL BASIS OF THE ECOLOGICAL PERSPECTIVE

How we deal with levels of analysis depends, in part, on our epistemological assumptions. The dominant logical positivistic paradigm—which emphasizes not only control but determinism, linear causality, and establishing the "truth" of preformulated propositions—does not require us to consider context. The logic of the paradigm makes it quite acceptable to create simplified, artificial situations in which to study pairs of single-level variables.

It is time for researchers in the relational psychologies to take seriously—to the point of application—the various challenges and alternatives to positivism that have been proposed (e.g., Blumer, 1969; Fiske & Schweder, 1986; Gergen, 1982; Lincoln & Guba, 1985; Wicker, 1986). Specifically, we should resist evaluations of research that are based on outmoded or inappropriate criteria. To take a single telling example, much mainstream research in social, organizational, and other psychological specialties is based on the following assumption: Data obtained from a narrow, homogeneous population of people performing short-term, researcher-imposed cognitive tasks in rarefied environments, are sufficiently compelling to validate hypotheses and to add credibility to universalist theories about human nature.

If we do not accept this self-serving assumption of generality, then we consider that research on people who are coping with important life problems in community settings is at least as informative about humanity as research on college students' thoughts about and responses to hypothetical or contrived situations.

THEORY UNDERLYING THE LEVELS ISSUE

Only a handful of theorists in the relational psychologies have thoughtfully discussed the levels issue; Shinn cites a number of them in Chapter 11. I would add Barker to those cited. Barker's contributions on this topic are well articulated in chapters on the ecological environment and on behavior-setting theory in *Ecological Psychology* (1968; also see Schoggen, 1989; Wicker, 1979/1984, 1987).

Barker (1968) describes nested hierarchical systems that are simultaneously interdependent and incommensurate, that is, that follow different laws. In his view, the boundaries between systems are, in fact, defined by the points at which different explanatory principles are needed. For example, the price of cattle in Chicago is linked to the movement of cattle trucks on Kansas highways, but the laws that govern one event are not sufficient to explain the other. Similarly, one cannot explain behavior settings completely by relying on the perceptions of participants. Nor can one fully account for the "life space" of persons by knowing the settings they currently occupy. Nevertheless, settings and the people who occupy them are mutually influential.

Among the implications for the relational psychologies that I draw from this stance are the following:

1. The person system and the surrounding system or systems should be analyzed in terms that are appropriate to them and not solely in terms of concepts from another level
2. Cross-system relationships should be explored, but researchers should recognize that the interdependence among systems is only partial.

To illustrate, school psychologists interested in students' academic performance should consider not only students and their teachers, but also such school-level events as staffing levels and curriculum policies. Staffing levels and curricula can influence teachers and students and be influenced by them, but such links cannot fully explain either the behavior of students and teachers or the school-level variables.

RESEARCH DEALING WITH MULTIPLE LEVELS

Published investigations that incorporate data from multiple levels are also relatively rare. More such efforts are needed, and journal editors and reviewers should be receptive to attempts to show cross-level linkages.

A large-scale survey of the literature on small groups (McGrath & Altman, 1966) provides some clues as to what may await those who attempt to link levels. The researchers examined 250 investigations to determine whether the research variables referred to (a) a quality of a group member, (b) a group, or (c) the broader context. An example of a group member variable would be an individual's feeling about his or her performance; a group variable would be a group's score on a task. Fifty percent of the tested relationships between variables at the same level (e.g., group member–group member) were statistically significant, compared with 32 percent of the relationships linking variables at different levels (e.g., group member–group). (These percentages are probably inflated, given that statistical significance is frequently one criterion for publication.)

This finding could indicate that separate systems such as persons and groups are relatively independent, or it could reflect the youth of our field— perhaps there are powerful cross-system links that we have not yet discovered (McGrath & Altman, 1966, p. 38). Other data from this survey suggest that shared method variance increases the likelihood of obtaining statistically significant results. Investigations that incorporate multiple-level analyses and that also use different methods for the different levels may "suffer" as a result. Researchers who generate higher-level variables from individual-level data may increase the chance of achieving statistical significance, but at the cost of using less appropriate measures. We should keep these findings in mind when we evaluate our own or others' cross-level research. For example, it may be appropriate to use a sliding scale in judging the statistical significance of findings, depending on the methods and levels of analysis used in the research (McGrath & Altman, 1966, p. 39).

METHODOLOGICAL RECOMMENDATIONS

My strongest advice in the methodological domain would be for us to reject what I call the "tyranny of the hypothesis"—the presumption (from the logical positivist paradigm) that no investigation should proceed unless the researcher is testing a preformulated hypothesis. Although it is certainly advisable to give some prior thought to what might be happening in a particular setting to be investigated, it is often premature to narrow one's focus to the relatively few variables captured by a hypothesis. We must broaden our conception of research to include investigations that develop theory and that, for example, have hypotheses as their product (cf. Blumer, 1969, Chap. 2).

We also can gain from examining and considering strategies used by other disciplines: sociology, anthropology, program evaluation, organizational behavior, nursing and education. These fields have explicitly or implicitly dealt with the levels-of-analysis issue and have developed some ways of addressing it.

RECOMMENDED ACTIONS FOR THE SCHOLARLY COMMUNITY

As teachers, researchers, writers, reviewers, and editors, we need to sensitize others to the importance of the levels-of-analysis issue and to promote work that addresses it.

This course of action can be pursued in several ways:

1. We should develop courses or seminars that deal explicitly with the problem-formulation side of the research process and that explore alternatives to traditional methodologies, including qualitative and historical research (cf. Taylor & Bogdan, 1984).

2. We should introduce epistemological issues into our substantive or "content" courses. We should make explicit the predominant assumptions of the field, show how they have structured our knowledge base, and consider alternative perspectives, including ones from beyond our own discipline.
3. We should look for ways to incorporate creativity and unorthodox procedures—including cross-level and longitudinal designs—in our own research and encourage others to do the same (cf. Wicker, 1985).

More generally, we should work to develop truly *relational* psychologies—including a community psychology worthy of the name.

B. A DEVELOPMENTAL PERSPECTIVE ON MULTIPLE LEVELS OF ANALYSIS IN COMMUNITY RESEARCH

LaRUE ALLEN

Understanding the complexity of the lives of children and adolescents, particularly those from high-risk families and communities, who are most likely to be in need of preventive or remedial mental-health intervention, requires research conceptualizations that are equally complex. Thus, the marriage of developmental and community psychology theory in addressing questions about children's lives as these lives are acted out across different levels of analysis is a timely one. Its timeliness does not, however, minimize the amount of upheaval and change that such a marriage will evoke among researchers who, although highly motivated, may be ill-prepared to confront theoretical integration on such a large scale. Developmental questions such as "What are the pathways to adaptive and maladaptive behavior for high-risk youth?" have already presented a severe challenge to our resources, with the need for labor-intensive and costly designs revealing how such processes unfold over time (see Chapter 4, by Lorion, in this volume). With the acknowledgment that the results of cross-level examinations can make a substantial contribution to a developmental understanding of phenomena comes the task of implementing research designs that monitor events vertically (i.e., across levels) as well as horizontally (i.e., across time).

A developmental approach to community research does not simply mean community research with children as subjects. Nor does it merely refer to research in which age is an independent variable. A developmental approach to community research begins with objectives such as "the promotion of competence in adolescent girls as a means of preventing repeated teen pregnancies."

Viewing such problems through a developmental lens involves becoming sensitive to matters such as these: (a) Developmental histories are needed, to provide important information regarding maturation trajectories, that is, how girls, or groups of girls, have typically evolved, and the path that their evolution is likely to take in the foreseeable future; (b) girls of the same general age may vary in their developmental needs and, therefore, respond best to different types of interventions; and (c) the development of competencies may be asynchronous within an individual girl (e.g., social maturity outdistancing cognitive maturity).

A developmental approach requires a great respect for time as an effect and for the fact that patterns of behavior are influenced by changes over time in intricate ways. Researchers who examine community phenomena through a developmental lens are always mindful of the fact that they are dealing with people in process—people with a history that is relevant to their current behavior, and people who are on a developmental trajectory that cannot be ignored, without risking failure to arrive at a complete understanding of the processes of interest.

Turning to the inclusion of levels of analysis in our developmental thinking about community research, I propose that the central issue raised is a conceptual one. How do we get a firm grasp on the nature, or definition, of an interaction of individuals and their environments across levels and over time (e.g., between teen mothers and the residential programs that provide them services)? Another way of asking the question is this: How do we describe to one another the fact that the relationship between a youth and a setting is more than a mathematical combination of the characteristics of the youth and setting individually and is a dynamic process rather than a static entity?

This issue has begun to be addressed in work done by Lorion, Seidman (1988), Sameroff, and others. Sameroff's (Sameroff & Chandler, 1975) transactional model endorses the ecological notion that there are reciprocal relationships between people and their contexts. Seidman has suggested that we call our focus on processes of people-in-context *relational constructs*. The addition of such a descriptive term to our vocabulary will allow us to focus on certain transitions and examine hypotheses that test this interaction, with a shared understanding of precisely what it is we are examining.

Within the larger category of relational constructs, there are exemplars that we need to identify, label, measure, and examine as processes. Examples come from the work of Bronfenbrenner (1979), whose terms *microsystem* and *mesosystem* are relational constructs describing different levels of analysis. Microsystem relationships are likely to be familiar to us, although perhaps without this specific label attached to them. Before there was a clear conceptual sense of the child–family relationship as a microsystem, for instance, research on parent–child interaction (e.g., Shinn, 1978) was frequently consulted for clues to the origins of maladaptive behavior.

The child–family microsystem is a readily agreed-upon relational construct. A child–residential treatment facility microsystem, although not readily found in the literature, does not violate our established ways of thinking. But the mesosystem relational construct, the relationship between a family and a residential treatment facility, especially considering the impact of that relationship on the child, is a new level of conceptualization, description, measurement, and analysis. Developmentalists such as Bronfenbrenner and Garbarino (e.g., Garbarino & Sherman, 1980) are embracing the ideal of varying levels of analysis in research, but struggle along with the rest of us in operationalizing this concern.

To continue with the example of the intervention program for pregnant adolescents, how might we capture the essence of the family–treatment program mesosystem? I would like to suggest that work on cross-level interaction (in this instance, analysis of the impact of a mesosystem relationship), whether involving one or more levels of analysis, will profit from refinements of our causal models that incorporate these interactions and their measurement as latent constructs. Our current approach to measuring family–program interaction most often involves taking measures of the family (e.g., its climate), and measures of the program (e.g., burnout and job satisfaction among staff), and then assessing interaction as a statistical measure of association. This approach does not require that we tap the relationship directly, and can therefore provide little data regarding changes in this relationship and the impact of these changes on our target child.

Our challenge, illustrated in Figure 1, is to focus on the interaction between family and program and the impact of that relationship on the child, Barbara. The traditional approach would have us look at family and program from Barbara's point of view, then measure the strength of the association between the two and assume that this procedure has captured the family–program relationship. An explicit emphasis on the impact of levels of analysis requires, I believe, that Arrows b and c in the figure be incorporated as mesosystem effects. Mesosystem measures, such as "frequency of contact," or "degree of cooperation/conflict" between family and program would reflect the family–program interaction whose

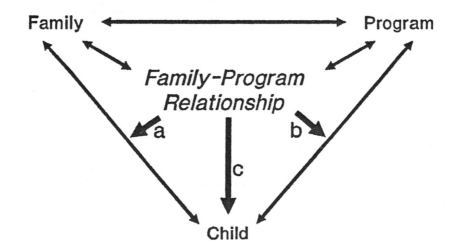

Figure 1 The relationship between family and program

impact on the child, through the child–family and child–program microsystems, would be assessed.

Arrow c is included as a discussion point that may or may not receive empirical validation. In specifying our model more fully through inclusion of the relationship construct, we are confronted with the theoretical possibility that the relationship may have a direct effect on the child, independent of the relationship's impact on child–family or child–program interaction. Here, the contribution of a developmental perspective is key, because only through the additional step of looking at the transactional relationships in Figure 1 over time can we define the components of the reciprocities in the model and discover whether the inclusion of Arrow c enhances our ability to capture reality.

The true nature of the task that I am proposing is a replication of Figure 1 across time, with time along the horizontal dimension and levels of analysis presented vertically. Evaluation of the interactions and mutual-influencing among levels of analysis becomes, then, a third dimension. We need consensual vocabulary and measures for getting at Arrows a and b, measures and vocabulary that do not degenerate into the depiction of behavior or attitudes at one level only, but truly reflect interaction. Once these mesosystem relationships are in focus, verbalized, and agreed upon, we can then monitor how change occurs sequentially.

Advancing this agenda, which demands the collaboration and close cooperation of those of us dedicated to finding solutions to this challenge, will increase our ability ultimately to promote the competence of people and settings, a major step toward realizing a fundamental objective of community psychology.

C. RESOLVING THE "MIXING AND MATCHING" PROBLEM: A VIEW FROM THE ORGANIZATIONAL PERSPECTIVE

CARY CHERNISS

The ideas presented by Shinn in Chapter 11 are particularly relevant for community psychology research and theory from the organizational perspective. In fact, organizational researchers have been more content to rely on individual-level, self-report or self-perceptual measures of the environment than have those in other areas of psychology, such as developmental psychology (e.g., mother–child interaction) or group dynamics.

An example of how the dilemma of multiple levels and perspectives arises in organizational research can be found in studies of supervisory behavior. Supervisory behavior (or style) represents a particularly salient aspect of the work environment. For decades, most organizational researchers were content to measure supervisory behavior by asking employees to complete paper-and-pencil instruments (Campbell, 1977). However, several studies have called this approach into question. For instance, Gilmore, Beehr, and Richter (1979) found that differences in supervisory behavior created in a controlled laboratory setting were not perceived by the subordinates, even though the differences were associated with significant variations in subordinate performance. In another laboratory study, Ilgen and Fujii (1976) found no relationship between descriptions of supervisor behavior provided by subordinates and by independent observers. Phillips (1976) obtained similar results in an in-depth field study. All of these organizational studies represent examples of the dilemmas that Shinn raises.

The dilemmas discussed by Shinn seem to be closely related to the epistemological issues raised in some of the other chapters in this book, especially by Riger in Chapter 5 and by Kingry-Westergaard and Kelly in Chapter 3. *Social constructionism* and variants of this epistemological view were developed in part precisely because of the difficulty encountered in trying to design objective measures of the external world that are independent of the biases of an observer. From the perspective of a social constructionist, the search for more objective, higher-level constructs and measures might be viewed as ultimately futile and misguided. Social constructionism implies that one never can design measures of the setting independent of the person, because the setting does not exist independently of the person. There is no absolute, objective setting out there—there are only many different settings, each a construction of an individual (or of a group of individuals with similar perspectives).

One implication of the social constructionist perspective is that subjective-perceptual measures of the environment are acceptable—in fact, desirable. Seemingly more "objective" measures are simply subjective-perceptual measures from a different vantage point.

However, Shinn identifies a problem that raises questions about the usefulness and validity of social constructionism. She notes that "aspects of the environment of which we are not consciously aware can exert powerful influences on behavior," giving as examples the influence of physical space or cultural belief systems that are taken for granted by members of a setting. If we rely on self-report measures of the environment, unconscious influences may go undetected. There is clearly no easy solution to the dilemmas raised by Shinn and by Kingry-Westergaard and Kelly in Chapter 3. But perhaps it will be useful to recognize that the main issues raised in each of these papers—the levels-of-analysis problem and the social constructionist challenge—are related in a fundamental way.

From an organizational perspective, one of the most exciting and potentially useful points made by Shinn is the suggestion that part of the problem is conceptual: We need new measures of the environment that identify more psychologically salient aspects, such as Barker, Gump, and Wicker's concept of *manning* or *staffing* as a replacement for size. In general, the organizational perspective has produced research that is rich in data-analytic techniques and relatively impoverished in concepts that are truly cross-level and extraindividual. However, there have been some notable exceptions: Role theory and open systems theory can, and do, provide some interesting attempts to develop such concepts (Katz & Kahn, 1978). For instance, the concept of the "role episode" provides a way of accounting for discrepancies between extraindividual ("the sent role") and individual level ("the received role") variables (Kahn, Wolfe, Quinn, Snoek, & Rosenthal, 1964). Similarly, the notion of *system boundaries* represents an interesting way of conceptualizing the discontinuities as well as the consistencies across different levels. Unfortunately, most researchers in the organizational behavior tradition, although giving lip service from time to time to these concepts, do not seem to be guided by them. Furthermore, there is almost no research that attempts to develop these concepts in ways that address the fundamental methodological problems raised by Shinn.

New concepts that deal with person–environment relations, rather than those that attempt to isolate "pure" aspects of the environment, seem to offer particularly promising ways of overcoming some of the methodological problems identified by Shinn. For example, returning to the problem of supervisory behavior, it might make more sense to develop constructs and measures of supervisor-subordinate relations that are truly relational or "transactional," as Lorion and Seidman propose in Chapters 4 and 9, respectively. Work on the leader-member exchange theory of leadership (Graen, Novak, & Sommerkamp, 1982) and leader-environment–follower interaction theory (Wofford & Srinivasan, 1983) represent some promising efforts in this regard.

Another interesting approach that has not been explored much in organizational research is to conceptualize discrepanices in perceptions of the environment as *measures* of the environment. Moos (1974) proposed such a strategy in his work on social climate, suggesting that discrepancies in the perceptions of staff and residents in treatment programs might be an important aspect of the environment. Thus, programs in which there was a high degree of agreement in staff and resident perceptions of social climate might represent one type of treatment environment, whereas programs in which there were large discrepancies would be experienced as very different kinds of environments. This general approach could be used in many areas of organizational research, and it seems to address some of the dilemmas related to doing research on multiple levels.

Triangulation is often proposed as a solution to the sorts of problems that Shinn raises. However, this "solution" still leaves us in a quandary. The underlying notion in triangulation is that one can be relatively confident about inferences that are based on multiple data sources. However, points of agreement among different sources may not be any more real than points where there are discrepancies: Shared agreement could be shared delusion. Furthermore, Moos's approach (described in the previous paragraph) suggests that discrepancies in perception may be more interesting and important in the long run than agreements.

One reason that there tends to be so much confusion between individual and higher-level variables in organizational research is that we typically rely on correlational designs, with measures taken at a single point in time. Given the difficulties involved in gaining entry to organizations for research purposes, this heavy reliance on correlational designs in understandable. However, longitudinal designs or field experiments sometimes are possible; and when studies of some aspects of the organization are designed by the experimenter in a way that can be specified with some precision, we have made considerable progress in teasing apart multilevel constructs. Fairweather (1967) and his associates have been calling for such an approach for some time. Perhaps organizational researchers should consider more carefully the possibilities of "experimental social innovation" before assuming that experimental control is impossible in studying a particular problem.

One final issue raised by Shinn that is especially timely for organizational researchers concerns the use of qualitative methodology. Traditionally, organizational research has been strongly tied to quantitative methods. However, there is a small but growing group within this perspective that has proposed greater use of ethnographic and related methodology (e.g., Van Maanen, Dabbs, & Faulkner, 1982; Whyte, 1948).

Nevertheless, actual published studies using qualitative methods are quite rare. There are few such studies to be found in the journals. One reason for this dearth is that many reports on qualitative research lend themselves more to monograph or book-length presentations. A second, more fundamental reason is the lack of recognized standards for the rigorous collection and analysis of qualitative data. Editors and reviewers have a well-established set of standards for evaluating most quantitative research submissions. However, they are on softer ground when reviewing a qualitative piece. Those who might consider doing qualitative research are aware of this fact, and they may assume that in the absence of well-established standards, their chances of having such research accepted for publication are diminished.

Actually, there are standards for evaluating the rigor of qualitative research. The qualitative tradition is weak in the field of psychology, but it has been stronger in other social sciences. There are several good works on qualitative methodology, and these could be the source of "standards for excellence" (e.g., Bouchard, 1976; Miles & Huberman, 1984). For instance, in his book on case study research, Yin (1985, pp. 140–146) identifies "five general characteristics of an exemplary case study": (a) significance (Is the material unusual and of general public interest?), (b) completeness (Has the investigator expended "exhaustive effort" in collecting all or most of the relevant evidence?), (c) consideration of alternative perspectives, (d) the display of sufficient evidence, and (e) presentation (Is the written report coherent and engaging?).

Four other standards of excellence for qualitative research worth mentioning include the following: (a) bias (Is the evidence presented neutrally, and whose voice is not heard?), (b) engagement (Has the researcher succeeded in becoming deeply engaged with the people and settings that are the focus of inquiry?), (c) multiple sources of evidence (e.g., observation, interviews, archival sources, physical artifacts), and (d) documentation (Has the researcher maintained a chain of evidence for each proposition that is made?). Without standards such as these, qualitative research will continue to be seen as "soft" and unscientific.

In conclusion, the ideas presented by Shinn are especially important for organizational researchers at this time. Despite their avowed focus on multilevel phenomena, organizational researchers have been especially guilty of the methodological sins so effectively highlighted by Shinn. However, Shinn's chapter should be seen as a stimulus for further thought. Until more progress is made in resolving the paradoxes raised by social constructionists and their critics and until new environmental constructs and measures are developed—including qualitative methods—problems associated with studying persons in settings may prove to be intractable.

D. GEE, BUT IT'S GREAT TO BE BACK HOME: MULTIPLE LEVELS FROM AN EMPOWERMENT PERSPECTIVE

WILLIAM S. DAVIDSON II

When faced with the invitation to be a "respondent/critic/advocate" to Shinn's chapter from an empowerment perspective, I was somewhat troubled. Having read drafts of Rappaport's (1989) chapter in this volume articulating a contemporary conceptualization of an empowerment perspective and Shinn's chapter on levels of conceptualization, measurement, and statistical analysis in community research, I was not sure that I had anything to say. Nor, save for reasons of academic lineage, was it clear why I was chosen to comment. I have learned to discuss such situations with my kids. They are typically a much tougher audience than my colleagues and often more sensible.

Hence, my "empowerment reaction" to Shinn's chapter is at least in part a function of a dinner-table debate, which I will try to summarize. I provided a brief description of the dimensions that characterize an empowerment perspective to my 12-year-old, "that's-not-fair" son and my 16-year-old college-algebra daughter. I described the multiple sets of rules and scripts that we admire in community psychology. I then summarized the multiple-levels perspective, reflecting on the dimensions offered by empowerment. The levels-of-assessment metaphor even seemed to make sense to my daughter. Yet she sensed discomfort and observed, "It doesn't seem like you're satisfied yet." My son listened intently, thought for a few minutes, and with furrowed brow reacted, "Sounds like your friends are confused. What are they trying to accomplish?"

CENTRAL DILEMMAS, CONFLICTS, AND TENSIONS

Before returning to the themes of confusion and lack of satisfaction, I want to elaborate on why these observations of adolescents rang true. In order to evaluate the empowerment issues of a multiple-levels perspective, a brief review of the dimensions of the field as suggested by an empowerment perspective is needed. To organize our thinking on this issue, I suggest a set of essential dilemmas that I believe represents the agenda that an empowerment perspective demands. I will further suggest that Shinn's chapter pushes several of these dilemmas toward resolution in very specific and useful ways.

The following paragraphs will provide a brief definition and explanation of each of the essential dilemmas. Many of these dilemmas draw heavily on the conceptualization provided by Rappaport in Chapter 6. It is, in fact, these conflicting demands, so characteristic of the empowerment litany, that have dominated the development of a psychology of the community. The final section of this commentary will involve a reaction to Shinn's key concepts.

1. The field should be problem driven (Fairweather & Davidson, 1986) and elegantly theoretical as well (Seidman, 1988). Empowerment demands that we focus on issues that are central to specific human concerns, yet it also has a rich theoretical history. This first dilemma juxtaposes two thrusts in the field that must be attended to concomitantly.

2. The field should focus on increasing our understanding of phenomena (Davidson, Redner, & Saul, 1983) and should also have action implications (Rappaport, 1977). As a field, we have long struggled to provide a true *understanding* of the social phenomena that we study, as opposed to merely predicting or controlling such phenomena. These are goals advocated by other areas of the social sciences. Yet many of the ethnographic-style methodologies that hold understanding as their primary goal have often been at odds with our action orientation. How can we act before we understand? How can we understand unless we act?

3. The field should focus on groups and constructs often ignored by the field and should be theoretically sophisticated. A major thrust of the empowerment perspective has been to focus on underserved or ignored groups. The goal has been to work for and with groups ignored by professionals and scientists in our society. Empowerment also suggests that we understand the social phenomena that we care about using sophisticated theoretical propositions. It is unclear how we can be theoretically sophisticated about issues and populations previously unstudied. The danger is that this perspective drives the field to be elegantly irrelevant or inaccurately practical.

4. Community psychology has aimed to support diversity (Ryan, 1971) and, at the same time, maintain experimental control (Fairweather & Davidson, 1986). A core tenet of the empowerment perspective is the value of diversity (Rappaport, Davidson, Wilson & Mitchell, 1975). An opposite pressure on the field is the demand for interventions to produce normalizing outcomes. Experimental rigor has often been synonymous with standardized outcome measures.

5. The field should be either passionately rational or rationally passionate. This dilemma is a variant of the old professional/scientist tension prominent in our history. A key ingredient in the empowerment perspective is the importance of being very involved in the social phenomena that we study. The clash of the roles of the distant scientist and the empowering partner require walking a narrow tightrope indeed. It has been argued that our real strength lies in our rational and scientific approach. Yet we have often disdained the social distance involved in the traditional rational approach and have held the furthering of personal or political values as important in our research.

6. The field's research methods should account for multilevel constructs and also for idiographic richness while assessing radiating impact (Kelly, 1971). These issues in many ways characterize the severe demands that the empowerment perspective places on the field and one area where Shinn's suggestions expand the boundaries. Empowerment adopted Kelly's (1970) earlier proposition concerning the importance of considering multiple levels of behavior. In combination with the call for idiographic richness, this dilemma places intense demands on our research methods. Our field has only a brief history of multivariate research. Many of our theories are bivariate. The goal of multilevel research that embraces idiographic principles is extremely challenging.

7. Research methods should attend to important aspects of the historical and current cultural context and should be policy relevant as well (Rappaport, 1977; Rappaport, Seidman, & Davidson, 1979; Sarason, 1972, 1974). This dilemma is closely related to Dilemma 6 above. It suggests that we consider the ecology of the phenomena of interest and that we speak to the policy implications of our work. Because much of our research has achieved neither, we have a lot of work ahead.

8. The field prefers longitudinal studies while it also seeks to examine the causes of change. An empowerment perspective views social phenomena as very dynamic. Hence, it is necessary to conduct studies longitudinally to capture the dynamic processes. The recognition that important phenomena are changing over time places higher standards on the search for causal relationships than has often been the case in psychology.

9. The field holds a conscious worldview that includes participants as collaborators and uses a language that acknowledges the strengths and positive qualities of collaborators. At the same time, we seek to address constructs that are relevant to multiple formal social science disciplines (Chavis, Stuckey, & Wandersman, 1983). It is assumed that this collaboration will be empowering to all involved. The inclusion of participants in the research process is central to an empowerment point of view. It is not only suggested that such collaboration is inherently valuable, but also that it will enhance each of the parties involved. Juxtaposed to our desire to communicate with multiple formal disciplines is our requirement to speak several "foreign languages."

10. The field should create empowering organizations that will create more resources, and at the same time, these organizations need to be local and small.

This dilemma characterizes the challenges presented us by the empowerment perspective. It suggests that we create small and local, yet powerful organizations. We have often thought of these as antithetical.

ADDITIONAL ISSUES SUGGESTED BY MULTILEVEL RESEARCH MODELS

As alluded to earlier, empowerment suggests the dilemmas above as a template against which to examine research in the field. As a group, these dilemmas present a very demanding agenda for the field. However, in many ways, Shinn suggests in her chapter that "this is not enough" and goes on to suggest three additional criteria.

11. It is important that the field examine multilevel variables and triangulate data-collection procedures as well. Shinn reminds us that any operation is inherently biased, and that truth is to be found in the consistency observed across method. Constructing multilevel triangulated research designs implies grandiose methodologies indeed. If we are going to have multiple variables, at multiple levels of behavior, assessed through multiple methods, the size of research projects will grow geometrically or exponentially.

12. The field's statistical analyses should examine both central tendencies and deviations. Our tradition in the field has been to search for explainable central tendencies. Shinn reminds us that our aim of examining, if not supporting, diversity demands that we also concern ourselves with deviations as a source of knowledge.

13. Shinn suggests that our research methods should include measures of both people and settings and should also avoid the potential confounding of levels of data and methodologies. Here again, we are encouraged to examine multiple levels of behavior, in a manner parallel to notions of person–environment fit, but are reminded that we often confuse the issue by mixing such levels.

14. Finally, Shinn implores us to push for new paradigms. It seems obvious by now that the dynamic complexity outlined by this position on methodology will demand new paradigms if our level of understanding is to parallel our conceptual sophistication.

I would suggest that Shinn's chapter, as it has expanded on the multilevel, multimodal aspects of the methodological implications of empowerment, ironically makes our confused dissatisfaction very hopeful. Her chapter outlines the beginnings of the methodological challenges that we face and suggests some new places to begin looking for insights concerning phenomena that we care about.

Related to this discussion, I suggest that we have returned to where we started over 20 years ago, regarding our lack of satisfaction with our level of understanding, involvement, and relevance. These issues are indeed exciting reflections of our beginnings and they constitute an accurate reflection of the state of the field. We need more discussion of them. Only by seeking to push back the boundaries of our conceptions and methods, as Shinn has done, will we advance.

It must be remembered that the unique contribution of Community Psychology to scientific knowledge is that these dilemmas must be wrestled with. Our challenge is to be aware of the complexity of the agenda that we have outlined for ourselves without being overwhelmed by it or assuming that all of its components must be realized immediately in every research endeavor. The optimism of the field suggests that these dilemmas will lead us to a unique understanding of the social issues that we care about. Gee, but it's good to be back home.

E. LEVELS OF CONCEPTUALIZATION IN COMMUNITY RESEARCH FROM A BEHAVIORAL PERSPECTIVE

MAURICE J. ELIAS

In 1977 Rappaport noted that second-order change is the product of strategies and tactics of intervention matched to the appropriate levels of analysis and action. He provided detailed examples of what he viewed as the four primary levels: individual, small group, organizational, and institutional or community. His writings challenged readers by clearly pointing out the way in which many problems that are being treated from a clinical perspective at the individual and small-group levels are linked to significant etiological or maintaining influences occurring at ecologically more encompassing levels. By focusing too narrowly on the individual and small-group levels, Rappaport argued, we condemn many of our interventions to "blaming the victim." Moreover, many change efforts leave the conditions generating the problems that one is attempting to address largely unaffected.

When McClure and his colleagues (1980) reviewed the literature on community psychology intervention, they found that Rappaport's caveat was well founded. The vast majority of research and intervention occurred at the individual and small-group levels of analysis. Yet the conceptualizations that accompanied the methodology more often reflected an ecological and systems perspective, including organizational and community-level processes. The mismatch of levels of conceptualization, measurement, analysis, and action appeared to be the norm in community psychology research.

In the previous chapter, Shinn has addressed the complexities and urgencies of matching "levels" in a way that extends Rappaport's earlier thinking to cover specific methods and research procedures and their implications. Among the significant sequelae of her seminal work is to point community psychologists once again in the direction of research and action undertaken from a behavioral perspective. For there appears to be a growing recognition that one must differentiate the concepts and procedures of behavioral-social learning theory—which capture and reflect the laws of learning and much of what is empirically and reliably known about human behavior—from some of the specific applications of behavioral approaches, which some community psychologists have found objectional (e.g., behavior modification in school and institutional settings; Bogat & Jason, in press; Fishman & Neigher, 1982).

The fundamental goals of community research appear to be understanding and action. These are, and have been, the goals of much work initiated from a behavioral perspective, as well. Given the long history of research and action undertaken from a behavioral perspective, there are some lessons learned that may bring to fruition some of the comprehensive suggestions raised by Shinn.

BACK TO BASICS CONCERNING HUMAN LEARNING

Behavioral research has contributed some powerful principles of human learning that are operative at all levels of nested ecological systems. The role of incentives and disincentives in human learning and performance and change is a basic example. A great deal of how people behave can be explained by the operation of incentives. To understand incentives properly, however, one cannot consider them solely as an individual-level variable. Rather, they form a construct that requires an analysis of within-level and across-level contingencies in the present and a comprehensive social learning history of the operation of various reinforcement schedules in the past. One illustration is how organizational and professional incentives operate to influence the behavior of researchers, often in a way that would be unpredictable from a focus only on their personal or familial incentives and disincentives.

Another example of a finding from the social learning area is the pervasiveness of escape and avoidance reactions in the face of actual or perceived difficulty. Rotter (1954) made it quite clear that avoidance was a powerful human behavioral response, very much related to perceived goal strength and attainability in a particular situation. In some writings in community psychology, it is tacitly assumed that a population receiving a program or experiencing a problem is interested in positive and proactive change. This, however, is a matter for empirical investigation, from a behavioral perspective. By adding a systematic consideration of the role of incentives, disincentives, and escape and avoidance tendencies when individuals, groups, or organizations are faced with problems, community researchers will be better able to account for stability and change at all levels of analysis.

A MORE SOPHISTICATED NOTION OF SITUATION SPECIFICITY

For many years researchers and program developers have confronted limitations in the extent to which interventions generalize as planned. The explanations for these limitations do not lie in the oversimplified person–situation debates of the 1970s and early 1980s. Rather, there is now a deeper appreciation of the configural calculus of interpersonal relationships and of human–organization interface. In the kinds of everyday phenomena and social problems upon which community and behavioral psychologists wish to have an impact, the variance is difficult to capture. Shinn (Chapter 11) asserts that conceptualization, measurement, and statistical analyses will have to incorporate a sophisticated notion of situational factors to produce any kind of breakthrough in the areas of community-related knowledge or intervention.

Interestingly, recent writings concerning the integration of ecological, transactional, and behavioral perspectives seem to hold much potential for operationalizing Shinn's ideas. Each of these perspectives offers parameters whose equivalence (or "match") cannot be presumed to occur across situations. From such a perspective, Shinn's point that community research and action involves multiple levels can be extended to include multiple contexts within levels. Depending on one's theory of the phenomena under study, achieving a desired change may require intervention at (a) one point at one level, (b) one point at each of several levels, (c) several points at one level, or (d) several points at several levels. Conceptualizations that include this kind of specificity will be more likely to lead to interventions for which transactional and ecological processes (such as ongoing networks of reciprocal relationships, and interdependence) will "carry" initial changes into what would be called "generalization."

Two research examples illustrate the value of considering both levels and contexts. Quattrochi-Tubin & Jason (1980) showed that reduction of television-watching in a nursing home environment was best accomplished by increasing interactions among the residents in a lounge area. The intervention was focused at one level of analysis—the small group—and upon two main points—staff–resident and resident–resident interactions. Behavioral-analytic observation and description of behaviors and interactions in the setting led to the choice of where and how to intervene. Interestingly, the intervention has multilevel significance, in that nursing home administrators were provided with an organizational-level strategy to attempt in other settings to reduce (passive) television-watching among residents, and some residents reported individual-level benefits related to self-efficacy and satisfying personal incentives to be helpful to others. This seemingly small study serves as an excellent example of the potency of the eco-transactional behavioral perspective for advancing the progress of community research and action toward the multilevel, setting-sensitive sophistication that Shinn believes is essential.

Organizations also provide changing contexts over time. A study of the process of children's transition to middle school began with a behaviorally based analysis of the various tasks that incoming children would be required to master. Information was solicited from teachers, administrators, special educators, and children. Several classes of tasks were identified, including establishing satisfactory peer relationships, coping with conflict with authority figures, negotiating academic demands, and mastering the logistics of the new building and routines. Most relevant for our current discussion is that the analyses revealed that the tasks occurred in several waves. Immediately upon entry into middle school, logistic concerns predominated. Throughout the first year, the remaining tasks listed earlier were relevant. However, at the end of the first year, a new task emerged: coping with pressures from older students to smoke, drink alcohol, or take drugs (Elias, Gara, & Ubriaco, 1985). Although a traditional use of these data might lead to individual and small-group-level interventions, it is clear from a community psychology perspective that organizational-level modification of middle-school practices might be essential for second-order change; such change would also ultimately incorporate behaviors at the small-group and individual levels. Equally clearly, neglecting the transactional nature of the middle-school environment at all levels would reduce the likelihood that an intervention at any one level or context will endure.

TECHNOLOGIES FOR MEASURING MULTILEVEL PROCESSES

Community psychology has placed great emphasis on process. One major address in the field was even titled, "It Ain't What You Do, It's the Way You Do It" (Kelly, 1979b). Processes that extend across levels and across settings and, in the context of intervention efforts, processes that also extend over time, must be carefully conceptualized and then represented in operational (or at least reliable and consensual) terms. How will this be done? When behavioral psychologists began to tackle the problem of treating families in crisis, they faced the task of analyzing the contingencies and other behavior parameters of individuals, dyads, families, and the environments in which families functioned. They made extensive use of techniques like interactional coding, event and behavior sampling, response class matrices, and time series approaches (Jason, 1989). A variety of innovative designs to measure setting-specific, low-intervention effects have been used in behavioral research, with much relevance for the kind of methods that Shinn advocates for community psychology (Barlow, Hayes, & Nelson, 1984).

PARSIMONY BY EMPHASIZING FUNCTIONAL RELATIONSHIPS

In defining community research as primarily cross-level, Shinn (Chapter 11), is implicitly acknowledging that many variables must be considered when investigating a phenomenon. Behavioral psychologists have emphasized the concept of *functional relationships* as a simplification strategy to represent a recursive and configural reality parsimoniously. What are the key variables and key relationships—regardless of level—that seem to be of greatest functional importance to the phenomena in question? A serious application of ecological and systems perspectives indicates that by affecting key aspects of interdependent systems, one can effect broad-based change. Such strategies are successfully exemplified in community-level preventive interventions by Perry and Jessor (1985) and Fawcett, Seekins, and Jason (1987). For years, concepts such as behavior chains and sequences, linked with discriminative stimuli and reinforcers, have been a part of behavioral methods. Joining such procedures with multilevel eco-transactional theory should help both behavioral and community psychologists to select more salient functional relationships as the focus of change efforts.

In conclusion, the behavioral perspective is rooted in a tradition of research and action and, as such, has a great deal to contribute to the developing multilevel perspective of community psychology, particularly as delineated by Shinn in Chapter 11. There is inherent compatibility in many areas, and behavioral research and intervention can inform discussions of levels of conceptualization, measurement, and statistical analysis in community research and action.

CHAPTER 13

CRITERIA OF EXCELLENCE III. METHODS OF STUDYING COMMUNITY PSYCHOLOGY

A. TOWARD EXCELLENCE IN QUANTITATIVE COMMUNITY RESEARCH

BRUCE D. RAPKIN AND EDWARD P. MULVEY

Quantitative methods are not really the "stuff" of community psychology. This is not because they are not used. On the contrary, community psychologists have used multivariate techniques in general use by social scientists and have been quite open to new methods, from factor analysis to multivariate analysis of variance to structural modeling. Moreover, it is not that these methods are scorned. When we evaluate the meaning of results or the quality of research, we value the standards of rigor that quantitative methods offer and imply. However, we are largely borrowers of quantitative approaches developed by other disciplines or areas of psychology. Consequently, data analysis often means finding the "right" quantitative tool in one or another statistical package. Community psychology has not directly contributed to the contents of the toolbox, nor have community psychologists critically appraised the "specs" of the tools that we use in terms of their appropriateness for our tasks.

This borrower's approach to quantitative methods has had subtle effects on the design of much community research. Although we intend to address complex relationships among behavior, attitudes, and abstract community structures, we are often in the position of reducing these issues to manageable chunks of research, using more or less standard methodological designs. In the name of empirical rigor, we trim the question, trying to stop short of making it trivial. As a result, rather than freeing us to ask the questions we choose, quantitative techniques often impose restrictions on the types of questions to be asked, restrictions that we accept for the sake of the obligatory data analysis that legitimizes our research. In short, we have often let statistical techniques determine how we think, and thus constrain what we do, without examining whether those constraints are necessary or desirable.

Our challenge here is to provide principles for assessing quantitative and methodological excellence in community research. To do this, we have placed the values and commitment to social action that define community psychology first and foremost. From this vantage, we have been able to identify ways in which accepted methodological traditions and assumptions are inconsistent with the values and goals that community psychology espouses. The six principles that we propose highlight some of these inconsistencies and point to some alternative quantitative approaches that may be more congruent with the goals of community research. The principles and action steps that we recommend reflect our belief that further progress in the field rests heavily on making quantitative methods the "stuff" of community psychology.

RECOMMENDED PRINCIPLES

Principle 1: Community Phenomena Are Not Simple, and Methods Must Reflect This Complexity

Of late, our field has been concerned with identifying appropriate "phenomena of interest" as disciplinary foci (e.g., Rappaport, 1987; Seidman, 1988). Our first principle recognizes that whatever questions and issues come to the fore, we should not start with the expectation that they can be described adequately in simple or global terms. Framing research hypotheses about simple linear relationships in an aggregate or searching for the most powerful structural model may lead to more empirically parsimonious explanations; but these approaches may impose models that cannot represent the inherent diversity found in community life. Consider a familiar example: If the correlation between "spouse support" and well-being is .45, whereas that between "work supervisor support" and well-being is .25, we would generally conclude that spouse support is more important (given sufficient statistical power). However, this approach seriously blinds us to the potential diversity underlying these results. By focusing on simple linear relationships, we lose sight of the fact that there may be some individuals in our sample for whom supervisor support takes precedence, that each of these variables might be related in nonlinear and equally powerful ways, or that there are a substantial number of individuals in the sample who have well-being in the absence of support of any kind. The correlations provide us with information about the relative prevalence of certain associations in our sample. They do not provide information about the variety of patterns, nor do they describe the strength of effects for any given individual. By failing to flesh out the many facets of such complex relationships, we assure that our research reifies a truth for the majority while ignoring the many patterns of relations that actually exist in the ecology.

This observation is more than merely an idle call for more elaborate empirical models; it is a call for a different approach to framing the analytic question in the first place. This principle calls for a change of rules in the research game. Rather then setting up studies to find significant linear relationships and a subsequent small amount of explained variance, the principle here calls for the testing of multiple models in different sections of the same data set. It would make considerable sense to follow Popper's (1968) call to specify the universe of alternative ways that measures can relate and frame sets of hypotheses regarding the prevalence of different patterns of association. Without such an effort to formulate diversified theory, we are placed in the undesirable situation of treating the most prevalent pattern as the truest.

Principle 2: Our Methods Should Bring Us Closer to the Community

The quantitative methods that we usually use impose distance between the investigator and the phenomena of interest by causing us to spend relatively little time with a lot of people (or settings). The justification for this approach is that large samples measured on common constructs allow us to generalize to the population. However, the concept of *population* as used in inferential statistics may make only limited sense from an ecological perspective (Linney & Reppucci, 1982). Building a nomothetic knowledge base regarding community functioning may be an unrealistic expectation, given the broad range of sociopolitical forces that necessarily jeopardize the stability of any set of observations of these phenomena. An ecological approach requires a research emphasis on contextual dependencies, whereas traditional quantitative methods ignore them.

It is important that we put into research practice what our activist proclivities have told us all along, that is, that a meaningful portrayal of community phenomena in quantitative terms does not depend on maintenance of an "objective" distance or on generalization to some idealized "population." Instead, we benefit from adequate familiarity with the process that we are measuring. To distance oneself as a precondition or a consequence of quantitative measurement is to ensure a limited vision of the topic addressed. Quantitative community research must be able to emphasize description of within-person (or setting) relationships in ways similar to the techniques used in functional behavior analysis or idiographic personality assessment (cf. Kanfer & Saslow, 1969; Lamiell, 1981). Methods for portraying regularities in the changes in relationships over time in a particular setting can provide valuable information without relying on an artificial or idealized external comparison. Such an approach could produce a rich set of observations about the development of people and settings under varying conditions and, thus, provide a solid foundation for identifying general principles about the ecology of community life.

Principle 3: Yardsticks Change as We Use Them

The most fundamental operation in quantitative measurement is the assignment of scores to observations. Our methods depend on the assumption that scores are inherently meaningful and directly comparable. However, in community research, this assumption may not always hold.

Consider a psychological evaluation of an empowerment intervention. Although we might expect individuals to report greater control over resources, it may be that empowerment raises expectations among individuals who start with low expectations for control. With their sights set higher, such individuals might experience reduced feelings of control and, hence, lower reported scores. A successful intervention could look like a failure, without explicit attention to the possible meanings that underpin responses to the scale used.

It is possible to account for differences in responding to the same items by directly assessing what scale points mean to individuals (e.g., looking at the differences between scale points like *somewhat in my control* and *completely in my control* either with more behaviorally based referent scales or with semistructured interviews). With multimethod attention to scaling, movement along a given yardstick can be distinguished from changes in the yardstick itself. In fact, changes in the calibration of yardsticks (e.g., reframing, consciousness raising) may be the goal of many community interventions. In such cases, change measures limited to simple, linear movement in scale scores may misdirect attention away from the phenomenon of interest.

Principle 4: Validation Must Take Ecology Into Account

Issues of validity and reliability are as essential to community research as to other psychological areas. However, traditional ways of operationalizing these standards do not always fit with a community perspective. *Validation* is generally viewed as convergence of measures from multiple perspectives. *Reliability* is generally seen as agreement of measurement over raters, time points, or settings. An important aspect of these definitions is that they were introduced as describing stable traits. Trait psychology relies on generalization of observations that are presumed to be identical across observers and occasions. Ecologically oriented investigations, however, require locating events in their specific physical, temporal, and relational contexts. Therefore, there is a tension between "psychometric soundness" in the traditional sense, and the ecological sensitivity of a measure: Measures may achieve stability and consistency by sacrificing the ability to detect this ecological variability. Mechanical reporting of reliability and validity indices devoid of information about the context in which coefficients were obtained misleads the ecologically minded researcher.

For community psychology, evidence for validity and reliability can best be evaluated in the theoretical context of a research program. Cronbach and

Meehl's (1955) broad understanding of construct validity is quite applicable. Rather than mechanically looking for convergence of multiple methods, interrater agreement or temporal stability, we must specify how we expect our constructs (regarding both characteristics and contexts) to interrelate and to change and, then, observe if they do. Note that this recommendation calls for going beyond "ecological validity," in the narrow sense of observing behaviors in their natural surround, with measures appropriate to the context. Instead, it pushes for validation as an ongoing process of testing assumptions about how measures of a phenomenon of interest change as contexts change.

Principle 5: Subjects Should Be Trusted

One of the most fundamental constructs in statistics, and one of the most difficult to reconcile with a community perspective, is the notion of *error variance*. We use this term so often that it is easy to overlook its implications. Error means that some of the information we gather from subjects should be ignored as random, incorrect, or meaningless. The implicit meaning connected with such an assumption deserves reconsideration, however. For example, in evaluating interventions, the analysis of variance model that we generally use is based on the assumption that treatment effects are the same for all individuals. Any deviation from this group effect is considered part of error variance. However, if most people change a great deal, and a few do not change at all, is it reasonable to say the intervention worked in an unqualified way?

If we desire to gain a perspective on the change process rather than merely demonstrate the feasibility or potency of a particular intervention technology, then diverse patterns of individual change must be viewed as more than random fluctuations in data. An alternative perspective, more consistent with community psychology's worldview, would be to determine who changes in what ways. To do so would allow us to observe the different ways that interventions (or other conditions) influence individuals. However, such an approach means that we must trust the veracity of individual observations, rather than lumping them together and assuming that the truth will emerge from the aggregate. Trusting our subjects means having confidence in their self-reports and in our observations— enough trust to propose a posteriori grouping of subjects or measures to analyze natural groups and patterns of effects. This confidence can come from being close to subjects and understanding the yardsticks that they use to evaluate themselves and their world, but it rests on a fundamentally different perspective about what is important in research. Furthermore, measures and research findings can be "socially validated," by asking respondents to explain what observations mean.

Principle 6: Qualitative and Quantitative Techniques Are Complementary, Not Exclusive

It is rare to find researchers systematically integrating qualitative and quantitative approaches within the same investigation, but efforts to do so would surely enhance the validity of community research. There are several ways that qualitative and quantitative approaches can complement each other, as suggested by Principles 1 through 5 above. First, both types of data in the same study can provide the opportunity for using quantitative and qualitative information in an iterative cycle, with questions raised by one methodology being answered by the other. This approach lends itself well to dealing with problems of construct validity and to identifying changes in yardsticks. Second, qualitative research can make it possible to explore processes that lie beyond the limitations of any quantitative methods. Qualitative analyses may help explain so-called error seen in quantitative results (cf. Lidz, Mulvey, Cleveland, & Appelbaum, 1989) by providing an alternative understanding of the ecologies that we study. Finally, qualitative data can guide quantitative analysis of complex phenomena, by isolating cases or subgroups that should be treated as distinct for theoretical reasons.

With the advent of more sophisticated computer hardware and software for textual analysis, the manipulation of large qualitative data sets has become both more feasible and less idiosyncratic. Unfortunately, data collection using multiple sources and generally unstructured techniques (such as taped interviews) is often discouraged in community psychology because of our traditional belief in the scientific purity of numerical hypothesis testing. The development of a rich qualitative data base, however, is a distinct advantage where the aim is one of hypothesis generation as well as straight hypothesis testing. Such a data base is another set of lenses, one that often provides a better focus for particular questions. Rather than engaging in a classic struggle over which view of the world is "truer," community psychologists would do well to work toward integrating both approaches into research designs.

CONCLUSION

In writing a brief summary of a detailed discussion, it is possible to present only a "skeleton" of many complex ideas. Each of the principles proposed above requires further elaboration. However, many of the quantitative methods of conducting research according to these principles are already widely available. Such methods include cluster analysis to identify the prevalence of patterns in a sample (cf. Hirsch & Rapkin, 1986), scaling analyses to better specify our yardsticks (cf. Rapkin, 1985), and time series analyses for identifying behavioral regularities (Gottman, 1979). Other suggestions that we have raised do not require high-tech solutions.

Community psychology was founded as a challenge to schools of psychology that espoused monolithic theories of individual behavior, devoid of concern for ecological interdependency. We must decide whether research that is good according to the dominant models of psychology is the kind of research that we want to foster. The choice is not for less rigor, but for an articulation of what *rigor* means from a community perspective. Anything less will leave community psychology trying to justify itself as "good science" according to standards that are antithetical to its worldview.

B. TOWARD THE USE OF QUALITATIVE METHODOLOGY IN COMMUNITY PSYCHOLOGY RESEARCH

KENNETH I. MATON

Qualitative methods have a rich and distinguished history in the social sciences, although they are rarely used in community psychology research. Qualitative methodology grapples with understanding phenomena by focusing on their human meaning and by interpreting human experience in context. Thus, it relies more on language than on numbers. Qualitative data-collection methods include nonparticipant observation, participant observation, archival retrieval, and unstructured or semistructured interviewing of participants and key informants. Qualitative data analysis tends to focus on the discovery of key, emergent themes within observational or interview-based data sets (Glaser & Strauss, 1967; Van Mannen, 1983).

Qualitative methodology has much to offer our discipline, either taken by itself or in combination with quantitative methodology. The low rate of utilization of qualitative methodology in community psychology research is probably due, in part, to deep reservations about the reliability and validity of qualitative data, and, in part, to the lack of established, replicable methods for qualitative data analysis.

TOWARD A SYSTEMATIC QUALITATIVE METHODOLOGY

Miles and Huberman (1984) present a detailed account of their attempt to develop systematic, replicable methods for collecting and analyzing qualitative data, as part of their study of the implementation of educational innovations. Only a glimpse of their work can be provided here. From a larger sample of 145 schools, a stratified sample of 12 schools was chosen for the qualitative field study. An experienced qualitative field researcher was assigned to each setting and visited the site regularly during the course of a school year. Sampling parameters for field data collection were conceptually based on available knowledge of educational innovation and encompassed key actors, events, settings, and processes. Miles and Huberman coordinated the research endeavor and, partially on the basis of emerging findings, helped to guide the ongoing data collection by the field researchers.

Primarily on the basis of observation and interviewing, field researchers compiled more than 2,500 pages of transcribed field notes in the research. These field notes constituted the raw data of the study and represented descriptive accounts of processes, people, events, and situations involved in educational innovation. Miles and Huberman (1984) describe a diversity of qualitative techniques used to analyze the field notes systematically, to check on data quality, and to draw and verify conclusions. Techniques used to assess data quality included checking for representativeness, checking for researcher effects, and triangulating evidence across data sources and methods. For instance, if a certain implementation practice was highly valued by informants at a certain site, triangulation of data might involve looking at student test scores, obtaining testimony of teachers using and not using the practice, and observing classrooms using and not using the practice (p. 235). Such data-quality checks often involved additional data collection in the ongoing work of the on-site field researchers.

Techniques for drawing and verifying conclusions about variable relationships included matrix displays, ruling out spurious relations, getting feedback from informants, looking for negative evidence, replicating a finding, and checking out rival explanations. For instance, as rival hypotheses emerged from the ongoing analysis and review of incoming field notes, additional data were collected within and across settings to examine alternative explanations explicitly. (The reader is encouraged to examine the Miles and Huberman (1984) text for additional information about specific qualitative data-collection and analysis methods.)

QUALITATIVE METHODOLOGY AND COMMUNITY PSYCHOLOGY RESEARCH GOALS

Qualitative methodology has the potential to contribute to various community psychology research goals, including description, hypothesis generation, hypothesis testing, and social intervention.

Description

Accurate, naturalistic description of phenomena of interest represents foundational work in any scientific discipline. Furthermore, an understanding of the natural history of a community or social problem should contribute directly to the effectiveness of social intervention. A primary advantage of qualitative methodology in terms of description is its ability to richly depict the experience of participants, to identify complex behavioral or social patterns, and to delineate the multifaceted nature of the situational–organizational–community context in which phenomena occur. For instance, an understanding of the distinctive culture of community settings and populations (Sarason, 1982a), and of setting development (e.g., Gruber & Trickett, 1987) can be uniquely aided by qualitative methods. Careful qualitative observation and interviewing on the basis of systematic sampling of persons, events, situations, and processes should be an important component of naturalistic descriptions of phenomena of interest.

Hypothesis Generation

Hypothesis generation represents an exciting and creative task for the community researcher and, on occasion, can lead to a complete reframing of a research area or social problem. Open-ended interviewing, careful observation, and disciplined reflection are especially likely to generate entirely new, alternative perspectives when the qualitative researcher is able to put aside preexisting theoretical biases. For instance, given qualitative observation of a setting and in-depth interviewing of participants, the qualitative researcher can juxtapose multiple "frames" and levels of data to generate a fresh, context-based understanding of individual–setting interrelationships (see Chapter 11, by Shinn). Furthermore, interpretation of quantitative findings can be aided by the availability of qualitative observational or interview data. For instance, qualitative data that contain information about the ecological context and about unmeasured factors will help provide an informed, empirical basis for generating hypotheses to explain unexpected or complex results.

Hypothesis Testing
Hypothesis testing is traditionally based on the statistical analysis of quantitative data. The qualitative analysis of qualitative data, taken by itself, would not generally represent a preferred procedure for hypothesis-testing work. One exception might be when qualitative observation or interviewing is uniquely able to reveal a behavioral pattern or cultural norm whose existence is sufficient to disconfirm a given research hypothesis. Furthermore, triangulation of data from qualitative and quantitative methods to assess key research variables and to help establish relationships among research variables would very likely result in greater confidence in findings than that gained by quantitative methods taken alone. Although the expected benefits of increased confidence in findings must be balanced with time and resource costs, the triangulation of qualitative and quantitative methods holds great promise for expanding the explanatory power and meaningfulness of community research.

Social Intervention
There are diverse pathways by which qualitative methodology can contribute to social-intervention-based research in community psychology. For instance, the ecological validity and usefulness of program evaluation results will very likely be enhanced by qualitative observation and interviewing of staff and program recipients. Especially useful in this regard are qualitative data that enable researchers to examine unanticipated consequences of interventions and that contribute to understanding the individual, setting, and community contextual factors that influence program implementation and impact across sites. An alternate action-related role for qualitative research is to give voice to disenfranchised populations and diverse subcultural groups, by portraying in a compelling manner their distinctive life experience and strengths (see Chapter 5, by Riger).

STANDARDS FOR QUALITATIVE RESEARCH
The dearth of published qualitative research in community psychology may stem in part from the absence of standards to guide the conduct and reporting of such research. A number of general standards are suggested here as an initial basis for

discussion within the discipline. First, qualitative data collection techniques should be replicable and should be described in sufficient detail so that investigators interested in replicating a study can do so. Second, the sampling of persons, settings, events, and processes should be as systematic as possible. Third, the qualitative data analysis should be as systematic as possible, and the procedures used should be explicitly described. Fourth, the choice of specific qualitative methods should be appropriate to the purpose of the research. Different data-collection and data-analysis techniques may be appropriate for description, hypothesis generation, hypothesis testing, and social intervention research goals. Fifth, the results should be based on sufficient supportive evidence to demonstrate reasonable credibility and validity. Sixth, the results should be compelling and interesting. Additional discussion of standards for qualitative methodology can be found in various sources, including Miles and Huberman (1984) and Van Mannen (1983).

C. HISTORICAL AND INVESTIGATIVE APPROACHES TO COMMUNITY RESEARCH

MURRAY LEVINE

This section will center on the epistemology of historical, ethnographic (observer and participant–observer), and investigative research approaches rather than on a discussion of how to do such research. The research has a kinship with scholarly and creative work undertaken in the humanities. Levine and Levine's (1970) *Social History of Helping Services* is an example of work undertaken in this tradition. Ethnographic studies such as Dollard's (1957) classic work, *Caste and Class in a Southern Town,* and Whyte's (1943) *Street Corner Society* are additional examples. Goldenberg's (1970) *Build Me a Mountain* is a further example of work by a community psychologist describing the creation of an alternative setting. Much of Seymour Sarason's influential work (e.g., Sarason, 1976, 1988) is in the tradition of the humanistic essay.

Psychology has not given sufficient recognition to that research tradition, although all of us are more influenced by such research reports than one would judge from examining our journals. As a consequence, the epistemology, or the basis for the claims to knowledge of research undertaken in that tradition, is not well developed; nor do we have standards for judging the claim that a given piece of work is a contribution to knowledge. Research in the tradition of the humanities is designed to help us transcend the limits of personal perception and to extend our understanding of some aspect of the world by providing representations and descriptions of experience. Extended understanding means that concepts that we developed previously are justifiably modified or changed after exposure to a representation of another's experience.

The basic research instrument in such work is the human intelligence trying to make sense out of observation (Dollard, 1957). The human intelligence includes all of the intellectual tools and styles of thought derived from the research worker's professional preparation, as well as the worker's general education and skills. (See Sarason, 1988, for a personal statement with regard to many of these issues.) The professional research worker has an obligation, imposed by virtue of membership in a scholarly community, to examine the limits of inferences from generalizations.

Any effort to test the limits of inference from an observation may be termed a *control* (Group for the Advancement of Psychiatry, 1959). Controls that are based on the logic of research design are necessary to safeguard against cognitive biases that affect the ability to observe and report (Naroll, 1983). Controls that are based on social processes of social inventions serve to safeguard against research reports that capitalize on chance variation, or that may, on occasion, prove fraudulent. These social controls include attempts at replication as well as peer review and criticism (Campbell, 1988; Levine, 1974).

Any observation is a perception, and every perception is in part a function of the perceiver's perspective. Instruments designed to enhance objectivity may alienate us from the phenomena of interest, and quantification, although sometimes adding to the precision of description, may interfere with the communicative value of a given representation of an observation. (For example, what would be the stimulation value of a erotic passage whose key terms were expressed in quantities?) In the humanities tradition, the typical form of a report is the essay, and, at its heart, the essay contains stories or analyses that are based on concretely described human events. These "thick descriptions" (Geertz, 1973) turn a "passing event . . . into an account . . . which exists in its inscriptions and can be reconsulted." (Geertz, 1973, p. 19).

These events serve as defining images or as key metaphors for a concept. It is likely that every theory has such concrete models as necessary, intermediate terms between the level of observation and the level of abstraction (Hesse, 1966). The concrete example typical of case studies, historical works, and investigative reporting (Levine, 1980) helps to define boundaries for the application of the concept that the writer has asserted for understanding new observations.

Observations made through investigative and historical approaches are subject to replication and to disconfirmation and, thus, meet some of the requirements of a scientific approach. The hallmarks of scientific endeavors include the public nature of observations and a basic belief in empiricism. The requirement that observations be replicable reflects those hallmarks in that others may make the same observations when properly instructed on how to make them. Empirical values are reflected in the requirement that scientific propositions be stated in such a way that they are subject to disconfirmation by further observations.

Once we are alerted to a core concept and we have some good examples to help define the core concept, others will observe similar events and can examine those events in light of the conceptual categories, illustrated by thick descriptions, used by the original investigator. Kanner's identification of autistic child syndrome was based on a report of 11 cases (Kanner, 1943). Others were able to confirm his report, in effect to replicate his original observations, and to show the utility of the diagnostic category for prognosis, if not for treatment. The careful description and analysis of events at Love Canal (Levine, 1982) served as a model to organize observations for other investigators who became interested in toxic waste sites located in other communities (e.g., Edelstein, 1988).

Goldenberg (1970) collected some quantitative data for his study of the residential treatment center that he established. However, most of the data that he presents consist of reports of observations, descriptions of places and interactions, interviews, verbatim transcripts of meetings, and other documents. He also employed a project historian to record significant events in the life of the alternative setting that he created. The concepts that he used to analyze the creation of settings have broad utility.

Disconfirmation of hypotheses also occurs in research undertaken in the clinical tradition, even though the hypotheses are not stated with precision, and even though they may not be tested quantitatively. Between 1930 and 1980, the *American Journal of Orthopsychiatry* published 59 articles indexed under the term *childhood schizophrenia*. When viewed in five-year intervals, a normal distribution can be observed, with 79.6 percent of all articles on childhood schizophrenia published between 1951 and 1965. There were but four articles published between 1966 and 1980 under this classification. Eisenberg and De-Maso (1985) attributed the change to the loss of interest of workers, who began with a hypothesis of psychogenic causation, and a second hypothesis that the childhood psychoses could be treated effectively by analytically oriented psychotherapy. "As reports on the outcome of the psychotic syndromes began to emerge . . . the relatively limited gains from the expenditures . . . of enormous time and effort cast doubt on the value of such heroic psychological interventions and raised questions about the validity of the conceptual model itself" (Eisenberg & DeMaso, 1985, p. xix). The decline in publications reflected not so much a change in fads as a disconfirmation of two hypotheses that resulted in a decline in research based on psychogenic views of childhood schizophrenia.

Standards of quality for research undertaken in the tradition of the humanities are not well developed. The standards of quality should be justifiable. Those reports that achieve the standards should be more worthy of belief because they say something reliable about the real world. Such standards are important because they can be used as the basis for deciding what further research to undertake, what to teach as the conventional wisdom, what to accept for publication in journals, how to distribute scarce resources (e.g., grants), and how to evaluate research and scholarship for promotion and tenure decisions.

We can include among these standards the requirement that the work be well written and compellingly illustrated. A well-written piece not only communicates, but indicates that the author has a mastery of the source materials, a clear appreciation of the work that the researcher undertook, and an awareness of the limits placed on the observer. Levine's (1982) study of Love Canal was based on thousands of hours of observation over several years and on interviews and interactions with players of all major roles in the community crisis.

We can have some degree of certainty about the basic facts presented by a piece of research when there is some form of corroborative evidence, observation by independent observers, or triangulation through other observations pointing to the same inference. Documents serve as evidence of facts, although these can have their limitations. Levine (1982) is a good example of how to use a variety of documents in a community research problem. In her study of the Love Canal community crisis, she used hundreds of newspaper clippings, official records, minutes of meetings, reports, flyers, graffiti, and correspondence. She also used the New York State Freedom of Information Act to obtain documents that were denied her by scientists involved in evaluating Love Canal health research. She suspected political influence in the interpretation of scientific data and obtained confirmation for the hypothesis of such influence in the documents released under the freedom-of-information request. Depending on how they are stated, hypotheses can be checked against the historical record.

An approach other than domination by the statistically based alpha value about what constitutes a justification for a finding is possible. Shapiro (1983) notes that members of the Royal Society, the British scientific society formed in the 17th century, were empiricists who preferred to trust their own senses. They quickly recognized that they would have to trust the reports of others. Before the formalization of statistical reasoning, *probable* meant *provable* or having an appearance of truth, or it referred to matters that could be reasonably expected to happen. Shapiro says there was a continuum ranging from *fiction* and *mere opinion* or *conjecture* through *probable* and *highly probable* to *moral certainty* at the apex. Placing knowledge along this continuum was a matter of evaluating the evidence adduced, the number of direct witnesses to a phenomenon, the bias and interest of the reporter, and the conformity of the phenomena to previous experience or their failure to so conform.

In many fields of study, the present state of knowledge or the phenomena of interest are such that we can only do the best that we can to pin down facts. When we tell others what we believe those facts to be, how we observed them, what limits there are to our inferences from them, and what alternative explanation may be plausible, others can arrive at a probability judgment about the knowledge that we claim to have produced. *Probability* refers to a subjective state that is justified by reference to evidence. In the end, that is probably all we ever have.

D. ECOLOGICAL VALIDITY AND THE DERITUALIZATION OF PROCESS

N. DICKON REPPUCCI

This section focuses on the concept of ecological validity—a concept that is embraced by many in the abstract, but that has been actually adhered to by few. An ecological approach to the human condition has a long history in psychology (e.g., Barker, 1968; Bronfenbrenner, 1979; Lewin, 1943a, 1952; Rappaport, 1977) and has been endorsed by most community psychologists. However, ecological validity has been difficult to define operationally and, consequently, difficult to measure. Most writers have suggested that it combines elements of ongoing interactions at multiple levels (e.g., individual, family, organizational, societal) between a person and his or her changing environmental contexts over time. For many it also implies studying people in natural contexts rather than in experimentally contrived ones. For example, a study of jury decision making using college sophomores as the subjects, performed in a psychology department laboratory, would have little, if any, ecological validity because of the artificiality of the context and the inappropriateness of the subjects. However, there is no agreed-upon definition of *ecological validity*, even though Bronfenbrenner (1979) tried to provide one a decade ago.

Most studies that call themselves ecological are qualitative and descriptive in nature because designing an ecologically valid experiment is extremely difficult for both methodological and ethical reasons. For example, a researcher who wants to understand the unique consequences of child sexual abuse cannot randomly select two matched groups of children and then abuse one of them. Thus, few experiments that even approached the goal of having ecological validity have been possible. In contrast, the research of Piotrkowski (1978) provides an example of intensive observational analysis of working-class families that has much ecological validity but that would never qualify as an experiment.

To find professional outlets for publication of ecologically oriented research is exceptionally difficult, because the work is not methodologically rigorous under the usual canons of experimental research, often referred to as "hard" science. Because "hard" science has come to mean "good" science and is inexorably linked with certain types of experimental design and analysis, researchers have been discouraged from pursuing research that might have some degree of ecological validity, because it frequently involves multiple levels of analysis simultaneously—a task that is still beyond many of our accepted research designs and statistical techniques. Although this state of affairs has been gradually changing with the development of such statistical techniques as structural equation modeling and cross-lag correlational analysis, these designs have usually been rejected because they often require years of data collection, large amounts of financial support, and long-term time commitments—resources to which most researchers do not have access. Moreover, because those who do strive for ecological validity in their work soon learn that they will not get published in recognized and prestigious outlets, they tend to give up the perspective for research. Security and tenure are the rewards of productive orthodoxy.

But does truth reside in "the heavenly city of the 18th-century philosophers?" Sarason (1976), in an article that should be required reading for all community psychologists, replies with a vehement *No.* Yet science has become our religion in that only certain methods are acceptable. As Sarason (1976) points out, G. Stanley Hall started us on this trajectory at the beginning of the present century, and we have seldom strayed from the path. Yet innumerable arguments have been made that those who have pursued this path of rigor have too often failed to see the forest for the trees. Ecological validity promises sight of both the forest and the trees, and it is a goal that warrants pursuit.

At the Chicago conference that served as the wellspring for this volume, I was the facilitator of the group discussing the issue of ecological validity in community psychology. I took careful notes and tried to steer the discussion toward some kind of statement that would sound learned and scientific and could serve as a foundation for writing this short piece on ecological validity. What actually took place was a conversation whose essence was that we must get rid of the shackles of unquestioned application of standard experimental designs and statistical analyses and examine their fit to each task, much as one must try on new clothes to determine which fit best. Although clarity as to what these new garments might be was illusory at best, Stanley Schneider, one of the participants, summed up the discussion by calling for a "deritualization of the process and product of community research" as we currently know it.

Deritualization appeared to be a code word for suggesting that the standard format for conducting and reporting research findings on community phenomena is not adequate to the task. Community phenomena are extremely complex, multilevel, and often not amenable to statistical analysis. Thus, the centrality of establishing statistical significance in research is questioned. In 1886, William James questioned G. Stanley Hall's decision to make the *American Journal of Psychology* "too empirical" (Sarason, 1976). He was ignored.

Hall's approach, emphasizing method, became the dominant feature of American psychology. Not only was it viewed as the path to truth, but it also became the criterion for membership in the fraternity. As Sarason (1976) stated:

> James and Dewey "became" philosophers, less because of any "becoming"
> dynamics on their part and more because of the way Pope Hall and his
> cardinals interpreted the relation among method, truth, and salvation. Poor
> James and Dewey! Fallen from grace because they interested themselves in
> such devilish themes as religious experience, pragmatism, existentialism,
> the nature of inquiry, the social contexts of learning, school and society.
> (pp. 1075–1076)

Community phenomena are much more like the subject matter that interested James and Dewey than that which interested Hall. Likewise, they do not
lend themselves to scientific consideration if only certain methods are acceptable
as science. These phenomena must be understood in context, or the concept of
ecological validity has no meaning. However, if method and statistical analysis
are predominant, then studying these phenomena may be impossible—like trying
to stick a square peg into a round hole. Unfortunately, because the peg does not
fit, we too often decide not to investigate phenomena by other means because
they are not acceptable in the house of scientific psychology. We may turn the
peg into a cylinder in order to make it fit, but the peg is no longer the phenomenon that we originally set out to study. In other words, it has lost its ecological
validity.

An example may be helpful. A community psychologist has developed an
intervention that requires working with mothers and fathers as family units, in
order to prevent elementary-school children from becoming disruptive. His or her
plan is to work with one group of at-risk parents and children and to compare the
results with a matched set of parents and children who are not subject to the
intervention. Unfortunately, he or she finds out that most high-risk families are
not intact natural-parent families. However, because the intervention requires two-
parent families, all others are excluded because they do not fit this criterion.
Moreover, to obtain a control group, he or she has to get parents from a second
elementary school, which operates under a very different educational philosophy
from that of the intervention school. In sum, although he or she has now obtained
an appropriate two-group design to which he or she can administer standard
measures pre- and postintervention, the facts that he or she no longer has a
representative sample of at-risk families or that children's behavior may be affected by significant settings to which they are exposed, have been neglected.
Ecological validity has been sacrificed in order to meet basic criteria for an
acceptable experimental design. Changes that drastically restrict the usefulness
of any results have been made for methodological rigor.

Impediments to ecological validity are not easily overcome. One guideline
offered by the members of the discussion group was a strong plea for thinking
about our methods. *Thinking* is defined as the presentation of a reasoned and
coherent argument or description. This process is in contrast to what has become
an often unthinking acceptance of standard measuring instruments and research
designs that are inappropriate for studying the phenomena of interest in a naturalistic context with its inherent complexities. Coherent description and observation may provide more insights into community phenomena than studying the
same phenomena in artificial situations that are amenable to tight research designs
and statistical analysis but have little or no ecological validity. The major issue is
not whether such experimentation can be ecologically valid, but rather to state
clearly that other methods of analysis and investigation may need to be employed
in order to understand community phenomena.

Perhaps the best way to make my point is to examine the essence of the method used by Seymour B. Sarason—in my opinion, the single most important thinker in community psychology. The following excerpt is from an unpublished paper entitled "Learning From Seymour Sarason" (Levine, Reppucci, & Weinstein, 1989) delivered by Murray Levine on the occasion of Sarason's retirement in April, 1989. It is based on tributes collected from numerous colleagues and included in a memory book presented to Sarason at that time:

> In a well-written piece, the representation "rings true." The reader who has no previous experience with the events depicted or the concepts, comes away with a feeling which says, "Yes, that's the way it must be." The reader with some knowledge or experience with the situation depicted has a slightly different reaction. That reader might say, "Yes, that's the way it is." The reader with experience will say, "Of course, That's what I was thinking and feeling, but I didn't know how to say it."
>
>   If anything is true of the statements in the memory book, it is that the writers referred to the insight they achieved from one or more of Seymour's books or articles. They describe how they were able to use the concepts they found in Seymour's writings to make sense out of their experiences, or to use them in structuring an approach to a new problem. It is the hallmark of propositions that we wish to accept as worthy of the term *scientific knowledge* that they lend themselves to replication or to prediction to new situations. Giving due recognition to the possibilities of mass delusion, we can say that the hallmark of the validity of Seymour's research and conceptualizations, the product of human intelligence making sense out of observation, is the power of the concepts to affect others. The concepts and their presentation allow others to see the same ideas worked through in conceptually similar but phenomenologically different contexts.

In short, Seymour's work is good science, although it is not "hard" science, because it produces a high-quality concept that is ecologically valid. His work is reliable and replicable. It illuminates phenomena for others, even though it seldom if ever has an alpha value attached.

This description of Seymour Sarason's thinking is the essence of what I believe the members of my group at the September 1988 Chicago conference were trying to express in their discussion of ecological validity. They strongly endorsed the notion that community psychologists should concentrate on this ecological validity whenever they study any phenomena of interest. Such validity may be arrived at through multiple paths and methods. Truth does not reside in a *t* value or a 2 × 2 design. Encouragement, not disqualification, should be given to investigators who try to embrace less empirical but equally rigorous descriptive analysis.

E. PERSON–ENVIRONMENT INTERACTION: THE QUESTION OF CONCEPTUAL VALIDITY

STEVAN E. HOBFOLL

Community psychology has emphasized that people must be considered in the context of their natural settings. Indeed, the term *community psychology* underscores that the setting and the psyche exist in an interwoven state. Together, the origins of the two words in Latin (*communis*) and Greek (*psykhe*) mean *common* and *soul*. Perhaps, these origins poetically portray the flavor of what is meant by the term—that new soul that is created when individuals are placed together.

The issue of conceptual validity must be compared and contrasted on the individual and community levels in order to understand what is special about the "common soul" advocated by the community perspective. Clinical and social psychology have tended to focus on a problem or an area of concern. Examples of this focus include the study of neurosis and the study of authoritarianism. To explain these phenomena, concepts were formulated and tested. To the extent that they could shed light on the problem or lead to solutions, concepts were confirmed as valid. To the extent that they did not shed light or contribute to solutions, they were either rejected or they led to new, more complex explanatory frameworks. This epistemological method is depicted in Figure 1. As may also be noted in this figure, the variables that would be derived from the individual focus would depict and describe the individual (e.g., denial) or the environment as it impinged on the individual (e.g., mother). It should also be seen that it is not only the concepts that develop, but that the view of the problem also changes and becomes more complex as the way it is characterized evolves.

Community psychology has been similarly motivated by the call of problems in society and, similarly, concepts have been derived to explain these problems and alleviate them. The search for understanding immediately becomes

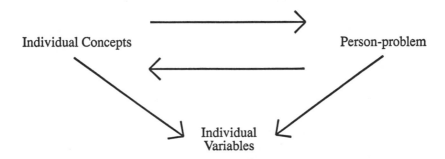

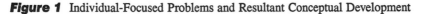
Figure 1 Individual-Focused Problems and Resultant Conceptual Development

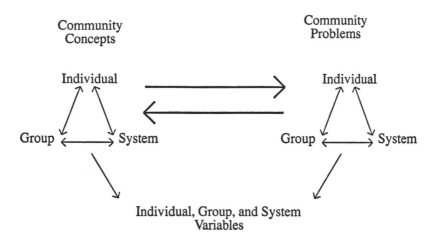

Figure 2 Community Problems and Resultant Conceptual Development

more complex for community psychology, however, because attention is given to individuals, groups, and systems. This enlarged field of concern is presented in Figure 2. Here it can be seen that we not only have individual, group, and system variables, but that we must also acknowledge the interaction that occurs between these levels.

An illustration of this approach is evidenced by the work currently in progress by Jason (1987) concerning intervention with children who are at high risk for educational and psychological problems owing to recent transfer to a new school environment. The program tutors individual children in order to decrease the likelihood of educational deficits. Group concern is illustrated by attempts to pair transfer children with buddies who will escort them through the entrée period and help them create and maintain their own support systems. The family group is also affected through family involvement in the children's adjustment to their new setting and home-based interventions to enhance adaptation. The systems level is included through teacher involvement and input, so that the interventions become an acceptable part of the school and not an outside intrusion into the teachers' domain. The greater school system is also involved, through coordination of the program from its inception with the superintendent of schools and the superintendent's staff.

What is striking both in Figure 2 and in this example is the complexity that a community approach uncovers. Like Pandora's box, once opened it cannot be closed. The complexity is a reflection of reality, and a return to the sanguine state of the closed box represents an incomplete and sterile forever after. It is instructive to look further at what is to be gained by this enlarged field of study. A sociological example might be helpful in this regard: Goffman (1961) and other sociologists suggested that institutionalization was a community problem that caused a labeling of individuals as mentally ill and a codification of their behavior. Conceptually, he presented the notion of the total institution as an explanatory framework that integrated the individual, group, and systems levels of this problem. This presentation also led to further theoretical developments, such as labeling theory. According to labeling theory, individuals who break certain social rules are assigned a label that identifies them as deviant. When this label is assigned to individuals, institutionalization and social reactions act to create career deviance from what otherwise may have passed as a phase or isolated instance (Scheff, 1966). Working, in part, from this conception, Fairweather (see Fairweather, Sanders, Cressler, Maynard, & Bleck, 1969), a pioneer community psychologist, developed a lodge program intervention. The lodge program instilled competency rather than illness-laden expectations in the day-to-day lives of mental patients, thus limiting the burden of negative labeling. It also adopted group notions and created cadres of patients who went through the program together and could offer mutual support. Begun on psychiatric wards, the intervention enjoyed only limited success. Thinking about the problem from the systems perspective that guided the project, Fairweather then revised the project to include continued work in community lodges (read *system*) following hospitalization. In the community, the process of reversing career deviance, begun on the ward, was continued over a prolonged period, until such time as the individuals were capable of release to more independent settings.

This example illustrates the importance of the complex individual, group, and systems interactions. Clearly, very different programs, conceptualizations, and discussions have been engendered from those of the individually focused view of mental illness. The example also sheds light on what the criteria for conceptual validity should be in community psychology.

First, the concepts should both aid in the understanding of a person–environment phenomenon and lead to programmatic and testable solutions to the problem. Second, concepts should be used as tools, and their value should be assessed by their contribution to solving or partially alleviating community problems.

A further criterion for conceptual validity is that concepts should engender new ways of looking at the problem and defining just what the problem of focus is. In this regard, our views and definitions of a problem are often naive and limited by that aspect of the problem that is unavailable to the viewer who examines the problem from a descriptive perspective. At their best, conceptual models provide us with a vantage point that is limited only by our ability to imagine. We can move forward in time, extrapolate, anticipate side-effects, and predict a probable course of events given intervention or preservation of the status quo. Without conceptual models, we can only wait and watch developments and solve problems in an after-the-fact fashion—we cannot describe what cannot be seen without conceptual modeling and theory development.

If any common theme emerged from the discussion of the working group at the September 1988 Chicago conference that considered the problem of conceptual validity it was this conclusion: Community psychology has as its raison d'être the search for solutions for problems that communities and individuals within communities face. This may be said to be the measuring stone from which any criterion for conceptual validity springs. Are initiatives being developed to combat the problem, lower its prevalence, or prevent its incidence? We must periodically fall back and evaluate the progress that we are making in supporting healthy community growth and healthy development of individuals within communities and the steps that we are taking to eradicate "dis-ease" factors.

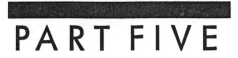

PART FIVE

IMPLEMENTING RESEARCH: TOUGH AND TENDER IN ACTION

CHAPTER 14

IMPLEMENTING RESEARCH: PUTTING OUR VALUES TO WORK

IRMA SERRANO-GARCÍA

> It is the participatory spirit of the research enterprise that carries it forward
> toward significant discovery, useful theory, and approximate application.
> (D. Klein, 1985)

Community psychology, as a burgeoning field, has been deeply concerned about research issues. How and where research is done, by whom and for whom, are questions that have pervaded its discussions. These are unsolved and unending issues, vital to a group that sees itself as creating a new discipline, a new look at reality.

The answers that this chapter provides to these questions will be greatly influenced by the particular social, political, and structural context from which it emerges. I live in Puerto Rico, a third-world nation beleaguered by poverty and the effects of colonization. This is a country where capitalism has failed and where democracy is weak. Our culture, composed mainly of Taino Indian, African, and Hispanic roots, is being continuously bludgeoned by U.S. values and customs. Our language is still Spanish, despite every effort to destroy it. Ours is an unstable country, where the roots of radical change are easy to envision and the hope for total transformation of our social and political structure is ever present.

Community psychology in Puerto Rico is of another nature. Its origins were separate from the results of the 1965 conference in Swampscott, MA (Bennet et al., 1966). It arose from a critique of traditional social psychology. Although the influence of the North American model of community psychology is pervasive in Puerto Rico, the influence of interdisciplinary thought is equally strong. We are continuously questioning influences from the United States and seeking links with Latin American and other third-world nations. Marxism, structural phenomenology, antipositivism, neopositivism, and social construction-ism are strong and highly valued parts of our everyday scientific life.

INTERVENTION WITHIN RESEARCH

Within this context, the quest for social change and empowerment is an essential aspect of scientific inquiry. Seeking these goals as well as ways to develop scientific knowledge, a number of colleagues and I have developed an approach that we call *intervention within research* (Alvarez, 1980; Irizarry & Serrano-García, 1979; Marti, 1980; Marti & Serrano-García, 1983, Rosario, 1984; Santiago & Perfecto, 1983; Serrano-García, Lopez & Rivera-Medina, 1987; Suarez, 1985). This model is a product of critiques leveled at positivism and is heavily influenced by recent developments in participatory research (Brown, 1983; Brown & Tandon, 1983; Fals-Borda & Rodriguez, 1985, "Special Feature," 1975). The overriding premise of intervention within research is that reality is socially con-structed (Berger & Luckmann, 1967; D'Aunno, Klein, & Susskind, 1985; Gergen, 1985; Hare-Mustin & Marecek 1988; Susskind, 1985). Understanding the constructed reality will require historical analysis to see how the phenomena of interest have varied across times and cultures. Reality will not depend on obser-vation and experimentation, but will be based on social exchanges, so as to construct, understand, and transform it (Gergen, 1985).

The research models and methods that we create must allow participants to express the categories with which they interpret and give meaning to their world and which lead to individual and collective understanding of reality (von Eckarts-berg, 1985). A new vision of totality. a multilevel approach that incorporates as many aspects of human life as possible in an integrated fashion, is required. It calls for the use of interdisciplinary information and popular knowledge. This approach is the focus of this chapter and, I believe, is the preferable guide for community researchers realizing their values in the research process.

Intervention within research considers research and action to be inseparable and simultaneous processes (Irizarry & Serrano-García, 1979), Serrano-García, in press). All action requires research, because human beings, while acting, construct and change their contexts as well as carry out informal kinds of inves-tigation. Research is impossible without action, because from the very moment that we start uncovering social constructions on reality we affect them. This means that it is equally important to acknowledge and to plan both the research and the intervention components of any study, taking into account their simulta-neity, their inseparability, and their mutual impact on one another.

We believe that human beings cannot be neutral (Howard, 1985). Not identifying or stating values is another way of supporting the status quo. Open expression of values facilitates the full evaluation of our work by others. It also allows the researcher to see how values influence endeavors, which increases his or her objectivity.

It is also indispensable to establish a horizontal relationship between participants (researchers and researched) in the process—a relationship of partners in change (D'Aunno & Price, 1984a; Keys & Frank, 1987a; Ortiz, 1985; Rappaport, 1977). We must acknowledge that the researched have habits, ideas, and values that are different from but not worse than ours and that allow us to learn from each other. This acknowledgment is an important step toward a collaborative relationship. The relationship that emerges should allow participants to share control of the research process as an instrument of their own development (Trickett, Kelly, & Vincent, 1985). A recognition of the community's potential to identify its own problems, needs, and resources as well as its capacity for social, political, and ideological development, is critical.

The developers of intervention within research believe that the primary commitment of researchers is to those people that make up the communities being investigated. This commitment should not require eliminating other commitments to science or to the professional community. However, if conflict exists, our priorities should be clear.

Many of the previously mentioned premises are based not only on a social constructionist view of science, but also on the certainty that a more equitable distribution of psychological and social (economic, cultural, political) resources is imperative (Joffe & Albee, 1981). In emphasizing the need for values clarification, a horizontal relationship, and primary commitment to community members, some of the basic notions of empowerment are being incorporated. The quest for empowerment is another basic ideological ingredient of intervention within research.

An empowerment ideology views power as a relationship that expands as more people have access to it (Katz, 1984; Lopez & Serrano-García, 1986; Swift & Levin, 1987). It includes among its premises the perception of people with many competencies and resources in continuous transactions with their environments (Rappaport, 1981; Trickett, 1984; Wolff, 1987). Other basic tenets of empowerment are the idea of change as constant, the perception of the observer and intervener roles as characterized by subjectivity and relativity (Swift & Levin, 1987), the need for a differentiation of diverse levels of intervention (Rappaport, 1977; Wolff, 1987), and a dialectic approach to the analysis of situations.

Empowerment is a process whereby people gain control over their lives, individually and collectively (Gesten & Jason, 1987; Gruber & Trickett, 1987; Keiffer, 1982; Rappaport, 1981, 1987; Serrano-García, Suarez, Alvarez, & Rosario, 1980). Contributions through research to the goal of empowerment have to develop a different set of guidelines. Those that have underlined traditional research have led it to become an agent of control within an oppressive and unfair system. It is toward the elimination of this oppression and inequality that our efforts are directed.

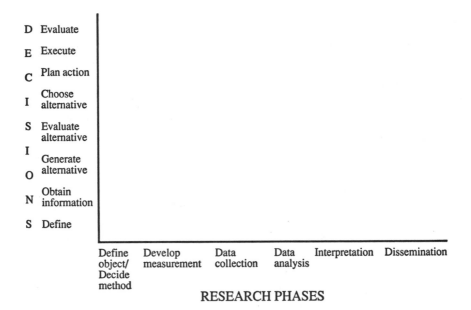

D	Evaluate
E	Execute
C	Plan action
I	Choose alternative
S	Evaluate alternative
I	Generate alternative
O	
N	Obtain information
S	Define

| Define object/ Decide method | Develop measurement | Data collection | Data analysis | Interpretation | Dissemination |

RESEARCH PHASES

Figure 1 Levels of participation in the research process

IMPLEMENTING OUR VALUES IN INTERVENTION WITHIN RESEARCH

The Horizontal Relationship and Participation

Participation is a central concept that serves as a means to a horizontal relationship among all research participants. We must begin by defining *participation* in contrast to a more frequently used term: *collaboration*. The *New Webster's Dictionary of the English Language* (1981) defines *collaboration* as "working together with others" (p. 197), whereas *participation* speaks "to taking part in, or sharing with another or others" (p. 691). It is my interpretation that *collaboration* as used in community research, denotes engaging the researched in executing the research, whereas *participation* entails their full involvement both in planning, decision making, and execution of tasks in the research process.

Participation is thus not achieved merely by allowing people to execute particular portions of our research, by convincing them of its usefulness, or by having them react to its results. Participation requires that we identify prevailing social constructions of reality and, in the process of doing so, create new ones. For this to happen, participants in research must decide what is to be studied, why, and how it is to be done. Thus, collaboration is included in participation but can also exist without it. When collaboration excludes decision making, the emerging relationship will probably be one of cooperation rather than one of equal control over the research process.

Figure 1 presents a way to envision the possible levels of participation of

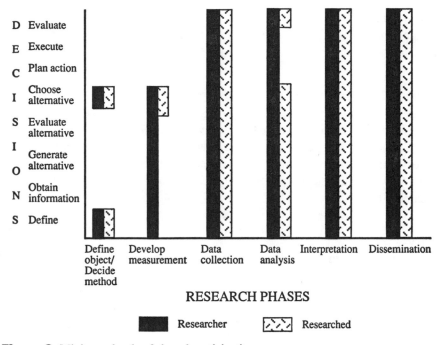

D	Evaluate
E	Execute
C	Plan action
I	Choose alternative
S	Evaluate alternative
I	Generate alternative
O	Obtain information
S	Define

Define object/ Decide method — Develop measurement — Data collection — Data analysis — Interpretation — Dissemination

RESEARCH PHASES

■ Researcher   ▨ Researched

Figure 2 Minimum levels of shared participation

participants. The horizontal axis presents the usual stages of any investigation. The vertical axis portrays the basic steps of the decision-making process (Brim, Glass, Lavin, & Goodman, 1962; Elliot, 1975). I believe that, ideally, all research participants should participate in all stages of both axes. However, such total participation is highly improbable, because research has shown that most people, when making decisions, delete various steps in the process, usually those that relate to generating and evaluating alternatives (Brim, Glass, Lavin, & Goodman, 1962).

The degree of participation needed to define the object of study and decide the data-collection methods depends on a variety of factors. First, factors that focus on the researcher include his or her paradigmatic position regarding research, commitment to participation and to shared control of the research process, skills and knowledge in concretizing these values, and institutional affiliation and the constraints that this affiliation generates. Second, factors that more directly concern the research are their prevailing attitudes and concepts about scientific inquiry, their levels of literacy and other "academic" skills, and the social–political climate of the community regarding their participation. A third set of important factors that have an impact on participation include the social–political climate in the society at large regarding participation and whether the researchers' entry into the community was requested by the community or solicited by the researchers themselves. Allowing for all these factors, Figure 2 identifies those areas where, in my opinion, participation should exist in order to achieve an equitable relationship that fosters shared control of the research process by all participants.

Entry, Continuation, and Ending

In order to specify ways to develop a participatory relationship I have divided the research process in three separate stages: *entry, continuation,* and *ending.* The examples and procedures that are presented here for each stage summarize diverse strategies that have been developed by different researchers in a variety of projects. Very few investigators have managed to carry out all the steps in one research effort.

Entry

This is the stage in which the basis for the research relationship is formed. During this period we, as researchers, must identify ways to share as much information as possible, to reveal our identity and purposes honestly, and to clarify all participants' roles.

Revealing information is a two-way process. How we go about it depends on who initiated the contact. If the community invited the researchers to work with them, they will tend to have much more influence on determining the object of study and the methodology to be used than the other way around.

Whoever has initiated the contact should promptly share the information gathered during this initial period. Sources should be revealed and data should be summarized, in meetings, in written form, or however else it may seem appropriate. To be consistent with the values of an integrated, multilevel, historical vision with an interdisciplinary focus, information should be obtained from archival data, from old-timers in the community, and from demographic, sociological, and anthropological studies (Trickett, Kelly, & Vincent, 1985). If this information has not been collected at the time of the initial contact, it should be gathered jointly.

During the entry period participants from all segments of the community should discuss how the setting has previously coped with and adapted to outsiders, how the local culture defines scientific inquiry, and how, according to current norms and practices, people participate in community affairs (Brown, 1983). Participants should also share their values concerning all these issues.

The research effort should be housed in the community. Its location should preferably be a place where people have customarily met (Trickett, Kelly, & Vincent, 1985). During the entry phase it will be necessary to establish a decision-making team for the project, such as was created by Bernal, Serrano-García, Alvarez, & Ribera (1989). That team included members of the groups or organizations initially contacted as well as people elected in community forums and assemblies. The research project consisted of three layers: the decision-making team (core group), the organizations, groups, or assemblies from which its members emerged (intermediate group), and other community members. A similar structure was established by Santiago and Perfecto (1983), who divided community members into two categories: data providers and nondata providers. In both projects the intermediate group was informed and consulted about project decisions in order to widen the community's influence on the project. Clear guidelines were developed regarding the nature of decisions entrusted to the core group and those that required consultation with the intermediate group. These examples have shown the evident need for an organizational structure that allows for meeting and mobilizing the intermediate group, or for other ways to consult them that do not require their meeting.

The core group, in consultation with the intermediate team, and if possible with the entire community (Santiago & Perfecto, 1983), should decide what problem to study and how to go about it. They should negotiate the purposes sought and share their commitments to sponsoring or funding institutions. In fact, if there are individual commitments to external groups or organizations, everyone should explicitly clarify whether they are negotiable, and to what degree.

It is important to establish a relationship of trust and honesty where the commitment to an equal distribution of resources within the research process is clear. The resources that the researchers can provide, such as time, consultative, or teaching skills, communication to outside resources, contributions to the maintenance of already available community resources, and creation of structures to facilitate participation (D'Aunno & Price, 1984b; Santiago & Perfecto, 1983; Trickett, Kelly, & Vincent, 1985) need to be specified. Similarly, community residents should realize the resources this kind of effort will require, such as time, energy, insight about community processes, communication efforts with different segments of the community, and willingness to learn new skills and concepts. In my experience, definitions of the roles of all participants—definitions that exclude the traditional roles of expert versus subject—emerge in this process.

Continuation
Belief in the social construction of reality acquires utmost importance during the process of measurement design and construction. The first task in constructivist measurement design must be the search for meanings and categories attributed by the participants to the object of study. Such categories can be obtained in the community through unstructured or focalized interviews (Colon, 1982), open-ended questionnaires, life histories (Runyan, 1984), or any other format that allows for unadulterated input from the community. Solano (1979) obtained the categories for a needs-assessment questionnaire by using the nominal group technique within community forums.

In other projects, such as that of Santiago & Perfecto (1983), final decisions regarding measurement construction were the result of a negotiation process.

During meetings with the core group decisions were made regarding which areas to include in the interview and which not to include. One major difference between the groups related to the inclusion of questions measuring socioeconomic status. The community group was strongly opposed to including these because they believed they would lead to divisions within the community. Despite all our "scientific" reasons for including the questions, based on the predictive validity of such measures, these questions were not included in the final instrument that was approved because community members could not be convinced of their advantage.

If in a negotiation process such as the one just described, participants agree to use predefined categories or instruments, evaluations and opinions regarding such measures are in order.

Researchers should also participate in this "meaning search." At this point, the use of traditional literature reviews is called for. Suggestions that emerge may include the use of valid positivistic techniques. A priori exclusion of any techniques, or the validation of meaning ascribed only by the community, would result in inadequate, "populist" research and the sacrifice of the considerable expertise available from the researchers. This model, far from rejecting traditional scientific knowledge, purports to enrich it through integration with popular knowledge.

Regardless of the magnitude of the entry process, in most cases large segments of the community will remain unaware of the research effort until the measurement and data-collection stages begin. Often another type of entry will be necessary to maximize the inclusion of people as data providers in the study.

It is important for data providers to be informed about the identity of the research participants, their institutional affiliations, and their bases of support. Furthermore, data providers should be aware of the purposes of the research effort, the potential use of the data, and the process that has already taken place. They should be asked whether they wish to provide the data requested and should be informed of what this provision implies in terms of their time, energy, and knowledge. Furthermore, they ought to be informed of any potential risks involved in providing the information. The confidentiality of the information should be guaranteed in as many ways as possible.

Participants should be consulted as to whether the reports that emerge from the research project may be published and as to whether they wish their community to be identified. Irizarry (1978) sent letters to all participants in his study asking them to state whether the results obtained for his master's thesis could be publicly presented and later housed in the university library. Fortunately no one was opposed, but arrangements had already been made to keep the thesis in a vault in the library if the community objected to its public use.

Finally, data providers should be informed of the means that will be used to provide them with feedback and to involve them in the development of future action plans. The above-mentioned procedures provide the research participants and the community with unique opportunities to explore responses to the research process and to generate creative interventions.

Ending

The final stage of the research process includes the analysis and interpretation of data and the process of its dissemination. If the previous stages of entry and continuation have developed as previously described, there should be a sizable number of participants and data providers that understand the nature of the data that are obtained. Santiago and Perfecto (1983) trained community members so that they could codify and tabulate interview results. Although this step implied a much slower process than would have taken place if computers were used, it provided for greater understanding of the research process and results. Interpretation, future implications, and action plans that may stem from the data will be limited to a few persons if all participants are not involved in some degree in the analysis.

Interpretation of the data should be done as collectively as possible. For example, the data should be disseminated in various ways. A written summary should be prepared and distributed in the community (Alvarez, 1980; Rosario, 1984). Community forums, workshops, or assemblies should be organized (Chavis, Stuckey, & Wandersman, 1983), starting with the data providers and spreading out to other segments of the community. One innovative example of this technique is the procedure developed by Castaneda, Domenech, and Figueroa (1987). They carried out a needs assessment of the homeless in Santurce, Puerto Rico. So as to provide feedback, they organized a group of homeless persons who designed collages with magazine clippings to present the research results to a larger group of the homeless at a soup kitchen. At the meeting, a group was formed to design further action steps. Not only were people informed of the data, but a leaders' group evolved from those that had been involved in designing the presentation.

People should be asked about their reactions to the data. Questions like the following should be included: Are the data consistent with your social construction of reality? Are the data surprising, and why? What do the data mean in terms of your social situation? Are there contradictions within the results? What have you learned about the object study? About yourselves? About your community? What changes should take place according to the results?

When these issues are being discussed, questions should be asked that place special emphasis on any contradictions that the data elicit: Why are the data not consistent with your previous constructions of reality? Does this mean there are limitations to research? Does it mean perceptions were inaccurate? Can the results be explained by looking at our social context, our social class, our ethnic or racial characteristics? Examination of these contradictions should lead to an increased desire for change and its pertinent goal setting.

Once this is done, community members should discuss future action plans. At this point, the researchers should clarify their commitments. Are they continuing in the process and accompanying the residents in future interventions? Are they providing ideas and suggestions and leaving the community to handle its own fate? Are they available for further consultation if they leave? The researchers should provide ideas for the creation of community structures and mechanisms that foster the continuation of community action.

Unsolved Issues

The suggestions presented previously are not devoid of difficulties. Some are:

1. The research process described above consumes much more time than the traditional research process. Efforts invested in maintaining the horizontal relationship between research participants and the "meaning search" that is necessary for measurement design are extremely time-consuming.
2. Community participants are imbued with the traditional ideas about research. Because of this, and because of the greater demand placed on community resources, they initially, and sometimes permanently, resist the degree of involvement that this method requires. In some situations the resistance is such that requiring their participation may become another form of oppression.
3. Most researchers are not trained in the use of this mode. Even when they believe in it, they lack many of the social, organizational, and political skills that it requires.
4. Institutions that employ researchers do not generally support this type of effort. Thus, the researcher may be risking his or her employment and status by engaging in participatory research.
5. Community requests for interventions will stem from different sources. Researchers must wonder whether the inviting group is minimally representative of community concerns, whether it will allow participation, and whether it constitutes a divisive force. If researchers are not invited to the community, should they enter at all?
6. The choice of members for both the core and intermediate groups is a difficult one. What mechanisms will allow the creation of groups that are committed to community well-being and empowerment?
7. Most of the data-analysis methods that are known to social scientists require an inordinate amount of time, particularly in light of the community's demands for prompt feedback and solutions. To compound this issue, we are taught not to use results until analysis is complete and thorough. Can methods be designed to yield accurate results in a shorter period of time? If not, what is the minimum of precision won which we would be willing to compromise?

We must question the support that this kind of model has within the psychological community and what interventions should be undertaken to facilitate its development. In my concluding remarks, I will turn to this last issue, that of a minimum set of standards and criteria that, according to the premises and strategies of constructionism and empowerment, should be used to evaluate research executed and published in community psychology.

STEPS TOWARD PARTICIPATION AND COLLABORATION

It would be illusory to believe that community psychology research will radically shift its posture to constructionism and empowerment. There are, however, already some indications of movement in this direction (Klein, 1985; Rappaport, 1981, 1987; Swift & Levin, 1987; Wolff, 1987) that are encouraging and lead me to believe that establishing collaboration as an initial goal for all community research would not be unrealistic. The suggestions that follow are guidelines for researchers who wish to approach the final goal of participation successfully.

For a collaborative relationship to develop, community research should take place in the community, not in the laboratory or the classroom. It should prefer techniques that foster community action and empowerment over techniques that foster individual action and atomization of communities (Marti & Serrano-García, 1983) and not depend exclusively on scientific literature for the determination of its object of study or on psychological literature for its justification. Evidence of other disciplines' contributions as well as that of the members of the researched community should be required.

Our definition of collaboration requires "working with others." Participants in the research project should jointly carry out the tasks and make some of the decisions that the task requires. Any publishable piece should describe the ways in which this relationship was constructed. In more specific terms, I would ask that all community research follow, *and report in publications*, procedures whereby the researchers.

1. Inform the community of their identity, affiliation, object of study, and methodology to be used;
2. obtain informed consent from the community where the research project is to take place;
3. guarantee confidentiality of information;
4. obtain the community's authorization for the publication of final reports;
5. involve community members in data collection; and
6. disseminate the data to the community when the research ends.

If these steps are taken, I am sure that other levels of participation will gradually follow. I have confidence in community members who will not execute tasks without being allowed, or guaranteed, some level of decision making.

The struggle for equality within the research relationship will continue whether we are open to it or not. It is happening in the third world, because in many countries the oppression exerted by those who control the scientific enterprise is more overt and deliberate than it is in the United States. If we wish to contribute to profound changes in our societies, we must foster joint control of science. Knowledge produced by scientists is not the objective description of an outside reality but the subjective creation of a social phenomenon. We must share control of science, because the creation and understanding of this social phenomenon will enhance our grasp of social reality and increase our communities' commitment to its transformation.

CHAPTER 15

CRITERIA OF EXCELLENCE IV. COLLABORATION AND ACTION

A. DEFINING THE RESEARCH RELATIONSHIP: MAXIMIZING PARTICIPATION IN AN UNEQUAL WORLD

MEG A. BOND

Many writers have criticized the traditional research stance, which places the researcher apart from and above those who are being researched (Brown, 1983; Serrano-García, Chapter 14 in this volume; Trickett, Kelly, & Vincent, 1985). These critiques have encouraged the creation of alternative settings that allow researchers and participants to work as partners in defining both their relationship and the work to be done (Chavis & Wandersman, 1986; Keys & Frank, 1987a). Much of this work describes the ideal research relationship as "equal" or based on "horizontal" or "nonhierarchical" bases (D'Aunno & Price, 1984b; Rappaport, 1977; also see Serrano-García, in this volume). But is such equality or lack of hierarchy really possible or realistic? Are we confusing mutual respect and participation with equality?

Although "flattening" the research hierarchy may be an ideal in community research, it is neither helpful nor honest to portray the roles of researcher and participant as equal. Some power inequality is inherent, and we need to be forthright about it. This does not mean being pompous or presumptuous about our role in research. Rather, we need to acknowledge the power and resource differences that typically exist and, thereby, accept additional responsibilities as researchers that are not necessarily balanced by parallel or complementary responsibilities on the part of participants. In our search for an equal relationship, do we run the risk of denying differences and mystifying the relationship and, thereby, end up being as oppressive as traditional researchers? This is the central question.

RESOURCE AND POWER DIFFERENCES

Several analyses of participative work propose that totally nonhierarchical participation can happen only when there are no differences in influence or in agendas among participants (e.g., Brown, 1983; Gruber & Trickett, 1987). Not only is such a lack of differences unlikely, it is not necessarily ideal.

Researchers and research participants have access to different resources that are critical to any research process. A relationship that is based on pooling those resources is of key importance in creating a valid picture of the community phenomena under study. However, whether researcher- or community-initiated, there are both differences and inequalities in the resources contributed by each party. The inequalities stem, at least in part, from differences in the types of informational resources, the participants' relationship to the information sought, and the investment in the work.

With respect to differences in informational resources, researchers typically have access to scientific knowledge, whereas participants provide popular knowledge. Although both scientific and popular knowledge are critical to developing an understanding of a phenomenon of interest, there is a mystique about scientific knowledge that leads many (inside and outside the research relationship) to value it more highly. Whenever one party has information that is useful but not generally accessible to another, that party has a degree of power over the other (French & Raven, 1972). It is only through the demystification of scientific knowledge that the research relationship can become equalized. In most research relationships that process of demystification can only be accomplished through the efforts of researchers. How can the sharing of information held by researchers and dispensed at the researchers' discretion portray anything other than unequal or hierarchical relationship?

Information becomes a source of power differences in the research relationship in another regard. Even if we as researchers share our purposes and preferences openly with research participants, as Serrano-García proposes in the previous chapter, the type of information that is relevant and appropriate for researchers to share is typically far less personal and intimate than the information that we ask from participants. Such sharing rarely brings a personal vulnerability equal to that resulting from the participants' disclosures about their lives. It is difficult to avoid some lopsidedness in the sharing of personal information in a search for better understanding of community phenomena.

Although the views in this chapter were stimulated by a discussion group at the September 1988 Chicago conference, they are not necessarily shared by the entire group.

RESEARCHER RESPONSIBILITY AND CRITERIA FOR DEFINING RELATIONSHIPS

In acknowledging these differences in resources and power, we researchers can begin to work toward a respectful, mutually beneficial relationship with participants. In contrast, by downplaying or ignoring power differences, we risk making it more difficult for all participants to confront inequalities directly or even to address simple misunderstandings. An unarticulated or ignored hierarchy has the potential, as the feminist movement discovered, to be even more oppressive than an explicit one that incorporates respect and avenues for honest and meaningful participation (Freedman, 1973).

It is with this powerful dynamic in mind that the following actions, constituting criteria for participation, are suggested as possible ways for researchers to facilitate participation in an unequal world:

1. Actively question or reevaluate what *participation* means in each new research situation. In order to avoid the presumption that involvement in each and every step of research is desired or valued by all research participants, we can be guided by the notion of person–environment fit. Each research situation may require a different version of participation that is based on the preferences, history, skills, and background (including race, class, and gender) of those involved. Researchers are responsible for ensuring a shared process for defining the style of research relationship (including type and amount of participation), which could also result in the joint framing of research questions.

2. Maximize mutual respect for the different resources each party brings to the research endeavor. Mutual respect does not imply homogeneity among parties, nor does it require the minimization of differences. In fact, it can be quite insulting to community members when a researcher tries overly hard to be "one of the gang." Developing mutual respect is a gradual process that is based on recognition of the unique resources provided by researchers and participants. The researchers learn respect for the community through involvement and observation, while earning respect from community members by sharing resources in a manner consistent with the community's culture and norms.

3. Recognize power differences while minimizing procedures that accentuate or rigidify a hierarchy. When researchers can work with participants during the initial phases of research to anticipate radiating effects of the research relationship, the power differences between researchers and participants are less likely to become oppressive or rigidified. For example, we can jointly develop mechanisms for resolving differences that emerge between individuals or groups during the course of research (Brown, 1983). We can also develop plans to give something back to participants (e.g., through encouragement, feedback, or ongoing consultation). Similarly, we have a responsibility to ensure that the process of our work does not simply reinforce the status quo.

4. Focus on the phenomenon, not on the person. Community research typically focuses on a social issue, problem, or dynamic within some defined

system. We work with individuals, but the focus is rarely on the person apart from the social problem. To the extent that we confuse the phenomenon of study with the person providing the information, we risk objectifying or depersonalizing research participants.

Emphasis on the phenomenon pushes us to understand the implications of our decisions as to who we question and where we enter a system for the purposes of research. These decisions should be guided by our theory regarding the social problem being studied rather than by the personalities or characteristics of particular participants. Clarity regarding what phenomena are of interest should guide our work. We should not allow the availability or convenience of a problem or population (e.g., psychology undergraduate students, people with mental retardation) to guide the questions that we ask.

In sum, I have argued that in developing a participative research relationship, we must openly acknowledge the resource and power differences among researchers and participants. In so doing, four actions constituting criteria for defining the research relationship at entry are suggested: Actively assess what participation means in each new research situation; maximize mutual respect while acknowledging resource differences; minimize structures that reify a rigid hierarchy; and focus on phenomena so as to avoid objectification of the people that are our partners in research endeavors.

B. FIDELITY AND ADAPTATION: COMBINING THE BEST OF BOTH PERSPECTIVES

ROGER P. WEISSBERG

Reviews of the literature on disseminating social innovations consistently highlight two major shortcomings. First, attempts to replicate beneficial demonstration projects in new settings generally produce less positive outcomes than the original effort (Berman & McLaughlin, 1978). Second, successful demonstration projects are difficult to institutionalize, and many that appear to endure often have difficulty sustaining their success (Hall & Hord, 1987; Rappaport, Seidman, & Davidson, 1979).

There is considerable debate among community psychologists about the best way to promote the effective adoption of beneficial social programs. This essay briefly describes two contrasting perspectives. According to the *profidelity* perspective, social innovations that are disseminated to new settings should be implemented with close correspondence, or fidelity, to a program developer's original validated model (Calsyn, Tornatzky, & Dittmar, 1977; Emshoff et al., 1987). In contrast, the proadaptation viewpoint asserts that the differing needs, values, and resources of new implementing sites require modification of model projects to conform to their idiosyncratic ecological contexts (Berman & McLaughlin, 1978; Rappaport et al., 1979). In this chapter, I suggest that community psychologists incorporate aspects of both approaches as they design and evaluate innovations and conclude with recommendations about priorities for future research in this area.

The research, development, and diffusion (RD&D) model of change, which is guided by a profidelity perspective, represents one potentially effective approach for creating and disseminating beneficial programs. According to this model, social innovations with well-specified program components are designed by "experts" who are familiar with the latest theoretical perspectives, intervention practices, and research findings. These programs are systematically field tested and validated before being disseminated to local settings. Then users across different sites who adopt validated programs are trained to implement them in a manner consistent with the program developer's specifications. Changing or diluting the program is believed to reduce its effectiveness as well as the likelihood of its continuation (Calsyn, Tornatzky, & Dittmar, 1977; Emshoff et al., 1987).

Proadaptation advocates challenge several key assumptions of the RD&D approach (Berman & McLaughlin, 1978; also see the previous chapter by Serrano-García). They point out that local adopters typically do not implement a program exactly as it has been designed. Instead they modify, or reinvent, validated demonstration projects to fit the needs of their target populations, service providers, or organizational structures. In contrast to the RD&D model that considers innovation adopters and implementers to be recipients of a packaged product, Serrano-García asserts that it is preferable to involve these individuals as *participants* throughout the entire process of establishing an innovation. Diagnosing needs, generating problem-resolution strategies, and selecting and shaping ecologically valid innovations to address perceived problems may all represent integral parts of the change process. Furthermore, stronger user commitment may develop from self-initiated and self-applied innovations. Thus, adaptation is likely to improve rather than devalue an innovation and to result in a longer program life.

So far, researchers have produced little data to clarify whether profidelity or proadaptation implementation strategies produce more beneficial outcomes or enduring programs. This failure is due, in part, to that fact that evaluations of social programs typically emphasize the assessment of pre- to postintervention participant outcomes while neglecting to measure the extent or quality of program implementation (Scheirer, 1987). Evaluators generally treat the delivery of a program as an all-or-nothing phenomenon rather than as a continuous variable. Doing so makes it impossible to specify systematically whether a program has been implemented with fidelity, to identify how and why it may have been adapted, and to relate critical program components or modifications to positive outcomes.

Dobson and Cook (1980) caution evaluators about the dangers of making Type III errors—that is, measuring the effects of a program that one assumes has been implemented properly, when in reality it may have been delivered inappropriately or not at all. For example, without assessing the quality of implementation, one may incorrectly label a program *ineffective* when, in fact, negative outcome findings are due to shortcomings in the delivery of treatment. Scheirer (1987) contends that it is preferable for investigators to begin program evaluations by adopting a tentative stance that an unclear innovation is being delivered in an uncertain fashion. Accordingly, prior to focusing on outcomes, a comprehensive evaluation should specify the program components that are supposed to be implemented, identify which ones are actually delivered, and measure how effectively they are delivered. Another critical task involves identifying social-system components (e.g., characteristics of the program deliverers, organizational variables) that contribute to the extent of implementation and the potential for institutionalization.

Recently, a few pioneering researchers have begun to develop informative strategies for measuring the extent and quality of program implementation (e.g., Hall & Hord, 1987; Blakely et al. 1987). First, they use systematic methods to operationalize critical program components of social innovations. Then, through structured interviews and observations, they are able to measure reliably the degree to which such components are implemented with fidelity or are adapted by program implementors. Using these approaches, they have begun to provide valuable information about how program implementation processes relate to behavioral outcomes of program recipients and to program viability.

As an illustration, Blakely et al. (1987) recently characterized seven nationally disseminated criminal-justice and education projects in terms of 60 to 100 specific program components that were evaluated as being implemented in an ideal, acceptable, or unacceptable manner. They also assessed the extent to which local adopters reinvented these projects by adding to or changing essential program components. Interestingly, program adopters were generally able to implement their programs at an acceptable level, and high-fidelity adopters produced more positive outcomes than low-fidelity adopters. In addition, local implementers who introduced new strategies to augment the effects of faithfully implemented components produced the most effective interventions. In other words, combining implementation fidelity with appropriate adaptation led to the best results.

The research of Blakely et al. (1987) and Hall and Hord (1987) offers helpful conceptual directions and experimental methods for researchers attempt-

Preparation of this chapter was supported in part by a grant awarded to Roger P. Weissberg by the William T. Grant Foundation Faculty Scholars Program in the Mental Health of Children.

ing to determine factors that promote the successful replication and institutionalization of innovations. It is likely that the nature of an innovation itself, the manner in which it is implemented, and individual- and system-level variables in an adopting site all interact to influence both the outcomes that a program produces and its viability. Given the availability of new approaches for evaluating program implementation, future research should clarify the circumstances under which a profidelity or proadaptation approach will produce positive findings, or when some combination of these strategies will create greater success.

RECOMMENDATIONS FOR FUTURE RESEARCH

1. It is essential that evaluators document the extent and quality of program implementation before reporting the behavioral outcomes produced by an innovation. Whenever feasible, relationships among these implementation variables and program effects should also be examined.

2. Future research must prioritize the examination of system-level variables and organizational structures that enhance or inhibit the effective implementation of innovations in diverse adopting sites. Community psychologists will be able to conduct better research in this area when they become more familiar with the concepts and methods advanced by the literatures of *program theory* and *implementation-process theory* (Scheirer, 1987).

3. More research is needed to identify factors that contribute to the successful continuation and institutionalization of social programs.

4. Profidelity advocates argue that the initial funding for social innovations should be provided to scientists to establish validated demonstration projects that would be disseminated with high-quality training to local sites. In contrast, some proadaptation proponents recommend the abandonment of the RD&D model in favor of funding organizations to build their local capacities to develop and to implement innovations. Perhaps funding long-term collaborations among scientists and local community settings as equal participants in the design (or adoption), implementation, and evaluation of innovations will produce the most beneficial programs that retain their effectiveness over time.

C. DISSEMINATION

ABRAHAM WANDERSMAN

According to the dictionary, the verb *to disseminate* means to spread widely, to disperse throughout, to spread abroad, as those sowing seed (such as ideas). We can easily ask ourselves the following question: For community psychology research, is there dissemination beyond such journals as the *American Journal of Community Psychology,* the *Journal of Community Psychology, Prevention in Human Services,* and the *Journal of Prevention*? At least since George Miller's "giving psychology away" American Psychological Association presidential address in 1969, there has been an ambiguous Rorschach-like stimulus for investigators to disseminate their work and knowledge. It is a critical part of the community psychology ethos to disseminate and to share research with citizens, consumers, and others (Heller, Price, Reinharz, Riger, & Wandersman, 1984). What needs to be carefully addressed is the what, why, and how of dissemination.

In relation to disseminating community psychology research, two major modes of community research can be distinguished: basic research and innovations or interventions.

BASIC RESEARCH

Whereas applied research (e.g., evaluation research) aims to provide knowledge that is useful for decision making, basic research "emphasizes the production of knowledge for its own sake and leaves its use to naturally occurring processes of dissemination and application" (Heller & Monahan, 1977, p. 74). Chavis, Stucky, and Wandersman (1983) provided an extensive discussion of the values and of the costs and benefits of disseminating basic research to the community. Essentially, they propose that, by disclosing what our results are and how we obtain them, we can enable the public to judge how to use them better. In this section, I will briefly describe some of the issues in disseminating basic research that they raised.

There are several potential benefits to disseminating research, both for citizens and for researchers. Basic research can be useful to citizens and community groups by providing citizens with useful information about the people or environment being studied, by providing exposure to the sources and ways of obtaining needed data and information (methodology), and by generating new knowledge, through the researcher-community feedback process, that can, in turn, be used by the community. The education of citizens about social science research and methods may enhance their competence and lead to their empowerment. For scientists, the direct and immediate interaction between scientist and citizen through dissemination and utilization of research results provides a feedback loop that refines the knowledge base. A synthesis that is critically needed in the generation of social knowledge is created. By communicating with citizens, scientists can learn more about their methods, the meaning of their results, and important future directions for research.

Some important practical issues to consider in the dissemination process include the resources and skills needed to disseminate, the extent of community and researcher control over the research, academic rewards and costs, and potential harm to the community.

Resources and skills. Working with citizens takes skills, time, energy, and personnel. Meetings need to be arranged and attended; clear expectations of concepts, goals, and methods need to be developed; and differences need to be negotiated. Many researchers may agree with the idea of utilizing basic research, yet few have been trained in the skills needed to accomplish this task. It is not suggested that scientists must now become practitioners, but that they should consider incorporating mechanisms for the utilization of knowledge in the research plan, such as the paid or voluntary involvement of practitioners, students, or volunteers in a utilization effort.

Control. When citizens become involved in research, the researcher may give up some control over the research project. This loss of control may generate added costs, because some of the original goals or techniques may be resisted by the citizens and changes may be necessary. These are clearly critical issues to a researcher.

Academic rewards and costs. What academic rewards and costs for utilizing research are received from colleagues, the researcher's institution, and funding agencies? Often, there appears to be little direct support from these sources.

Potential harm. In addition to these concerns, which were all raised by Chavis et al. (1983), a fourth concern in disseminating basic research is the potential harm to the community. Two particular sources of harm are unintended misuse of the information because of partial explanation to the community of the information's meaning, resulting in the basic information being applied beyond its capabilities, and unmonitored dissemination, resulting in misapplication and distortion in application of the information (P. Tolan, personal communication, January 6, 1989).

INNOVATIONS

Fairweather and Davidson (1986) provide an extensive discussion of the why and how of disseminating social programs that have been evaluated and found to be helpful. They discuss the phases of the dissemination process—approach, persuasion, activation, and diffusion.

The first step in the dissemination involves *approaching* the potential consumer. Personal approaches such as direct contact or indirect approaches such as media and mailings can be used. The method chosen can affect the extent and impact of the dissemination.

In the *persuasion* phase, the potential adopter is brought from a state of initial awareness (in the approach phase) to a decision about adopting the innovation. The attitude-change research components of style of persuasion, content of message, and legitimacy of persuader are important factors in this phase.

The *activation* phase involves the implementation of the innovation. Refining the integrity of the new program to its model while allowing adaption to the setting needs and to community involvement is a critical issue.

In the *diffusion* phase, some of the original target population has implemented the program and is involved in disseminating the innovation to others. The critical issue at this phase is maintenance of the program and simultaneous adaptation to the changing needs of the community.

When to disseminate research results is a major unsettled question for community researchers. Because there is no regulatory group similar to the Food and Drug Administration to certify the quality of information or programs to be disseminated, the ethics of dissemination must be considered by each researcher. Considerations include the following: What is the demonstrated utility of the project? Is the information or program likely to do harm? Who is responsible? The complexity of the last is exemplified by further issues such as who is responsible for a good product and what is the responsibility of the consumer, once the possible side effects are described and informed consent is used.

CRITERIA OF EXCELLENCE IN DISSEMINATION

Given these critical concerns, the following criteria of excellence in dissemination are suggested for developing and evaluating our research. The applicability and importance of each depends on the type of research (basic, innovation) and other specifics of the project. These criteria explicitly adopt Shadish's concerns (see Chapter 2 in this volume) about taking into account a plausible range of values so that one's own values do not dominate. They also should result in research having "constituent validity":

1. Was the dissemination part of the original conceptualization of the research project (so that salient consumer issues were part of it)?
2. Were the values of the program carefully looked at?
3. Was there a search for unintended consequences?
4. Where applicable, were people who held different values from the investigator or consumer population asked to evaluate the project?
5. Did consumers or recipients help evaluate the project?
6. Were a long-term follow-up and continuous evaluation conducted?
7. Was the program successfully replicated by someone outside the original research team?

D. DATA FEEDBACK AND COMMUNICATION TO THE HOST SETTING

W. LAVOME ROBINSON

Community methodologists in a community setting are, in essence, guests in a host setting. This characterization of the research relationship between community methodologists and community members clarifies that the relationship must be one of sharing, parity, respect, courtesy, and joint collaboration. As detailed by Serrano-García in the previous chapter indigenous community members have an understanding and a knowledge base that qualifies them to serve as equal contributors to the social construction of knowledge. In order to promote a joint effort, prudent protocol calls for attending to the nuances of the working relationship or of the research contract. Doing so means negotiating and delineating from the beginning such issues as (a) data ownership, (b) target audience(s) for data dissemination, (c) the timing of data dissemination, and (d) the commitment and assurances of the methodologists to those researched.

Within the conceptual frame of action-oriented and participatory community research, feedback and communication processes are operative at many levels, including (a) the design of the research, (b) research implementation, (c) interpretive analyses of the data, and (d) data dissemination. The design of the research begins with the initial contact with the host research setting; thus, from the start, feedback and communication processes are in effect. In participatory community research, the development of the research agenda is a joint endeavor between community methodologists and the host setting, necessitating that the research team consists of (a) individuals formally trained in research methodology, (b) community members at large, and (c) a representative core subgroup of the larger community, which enjoys constant monitoring and input authority in the research process. Participatory research design includes community input in (a) determining the questions to examine, (b) the selection of actual research participants, (c) the choice of measures to use, and (d) the establishment of the procedures to follow. In addition, intermittent and ongoing consumer feedback mechanisms are incorporated to permit modifications and refinements to the research process. This nontraditional approach to research design and the embodiment of the research team reflects the valuing of collaboration and promotes a greater flow of information between community members and methodologists. In brief, participatory research designs advance horizontal relationships between researchers and those researched (see Chapter 14 in this volume).

There are many potential obstacles, even for the most elegant of research designs, during the implementation phase of research. In this research context, issues of empowerment, trust, and understanding become figural. The consent and support of the community to the research process must be incrementally secured; it is not merely given. Community members, along with community methodologists, are key players in the logistical and procedural implementation of the research project. In order for procedural collaboration to occur, community participants must clearly understand the research process. The language used to communicate procedural expectations must be familiar to the community participants; at the same time, the language used must not be patronizing (i.e., overly simplistic). The appropriate choice of vocabulary and its connotations require a sensitive awareness of the population to be served.

Community methodologists are often perceived as agents of a system that has historically been oppressive and discriminatory (Gaernter & Dovidio, 1987). Understandably, community members question the ultimate use of the data generated by the research project. Disappointingly, researchers have some history of using data in a flawed and biased fashion. Two examples are the notoriety of the Jensen studies (Jensen, 1969, 1973) and the famous Clark and Clark studies (1939, 1947). Both portrayed Afro-American culture as pathogenic. Although later studies have criticized the interpretive integrity of the Jensen studies (Gould, 1981) and the methodological sophistication of the Clark and Clark studies (Powell-Hopson & Hopson, 1989), the negative ramifications of these reports remain.

At the analysis stage, communication is shaped by the choice of statistical analytic procedures and by the interpretation of the ensuing statistical findings. In other words, research findings are a function of methodological and interpretive procedures; any variation in these procedures may result in an alteration of the research findings. Typically, community investigators with formal training in research methodology choose the statistical procedures to employ, and they also interpret the statistical results. These actions are based on the assumption that only the experts (i.e., those with formal research training) are suited to this task (see Serrano-García's chapter). This may communicate an exclusivity to community members. However, by virtue of their experiences, those individuals who are indigenous to the community can help select fitting analytic approaches. This inclusionary stance (as opposed to an exclusionary one) is not only ideologically consistent and strategically sound—it is also good ethics. It is the ethical obligation and professional responsibility of community researchers to guard against any misuse and noncontextual representation of the data (American Psychological Association, 1982). This ethical and professional responsibility can be met by educating community members to the research process, so that they may serve as full collaborators.

The information-dissemination stage of communication entails making the research results and implications available to the community and to the scholarly world, as well as positioning the receptivity of both spheres to the data. As evidenced by the initiation of two journals devoted exclusively to community research (i.e., *American Journal of Community Psychology* and *Journal of Community Psychology*) and several books detailing community research in action (Karoly, 1985; Posavac & Carey, 1989; Susskind & Klein, 1985; Zautra, Bachrach, & Hess, 1983), community methodologists are adept at disseminating information to the scholarly world. Efforts to communicate and to disseminate research findings to community settings have been less than optimal, necessitating an examination of current practices and the possible development of alternative strategies. The receptivity of the community to the research findings is considerably enhanced when the community is instrumental in the design of the research. The community's input assures that the research is consistent with the needs and goals of the community; the investment in the research process and outcome becomes a shared entity between the community members and the research methodologists.

Receptivity to information by the community is also influenced by the method(s) of data presentation. Whether a community is receptive to the findings of community research may be more a function of the method(s) of information dissemination than of inherent community resistance. For example, the use of graphs and other visuals may be used to enrich the narrative presentation of the data. Moreover, the poignancy of the narrative presentation is augmented when the narrative is concise and sensitive; again, the vernacular used should be familiar and understandable to the community. Community investigators are encouraged to consider alternative opportunities for information dissemination (i.e., the media, mass, mass mailings, direct contact, and other communiqués), expanding upon scholarly presentations and journal entries.

The belief that the appropriate time for feedback is upon completion of the study (e.g., debriefing) and that feedback should be a summary of findings rather than a detailed accounting of the process as well as products may be too rigid and, therefore, counterproductive for community research. Although it is reasonable to limit information flow to avoid data contamination, this belief conflicts with the philosophical underpinnings of collaboration and the status bestowed upon invited guests. In recognition of the "guest" status of community methodologists, it is a "faux pas" to continually request favors of others without some disclosure of the activity's purpose and impact. To reiterate, the information-dissemination process must include continued and intermittent progress reports and feedback to the community. The idea of flexibility in the feedback process also includes an openness to communicate to the host setting apparent trends and observations that may not have stringent statistical support, as well as qualitative observations. A posture of sharing and immediacy in the feedback process solidifies a cooperative relationship between research methodologists and community members.

The feedback and communication nuances between community methodologists and community members are numerous and extend beyond those elaborated. However, the essential question is this: How can we best embrace and preserve the value of full inclusion of both community methodologists and those researched? The solution requires an openness to alternative and nontraditional research practices and relationships that value equal participation and contribution by all parties involved in the research process.

E. RESEARCH AS INTERVENTION

CAROLYN F. SWIFT

Research can affect participants' lives by intervention effects that are unanticipated and unintended by the researcher. A classic example is the "Hawthorne effect." In a series of experiments conducted at the Hawthorne plant in Illinois between 1924 and 1932, staff of the Western Electric Company studied changes in workers' productivity related to changes in their work environment. The surprising outcome was that, although productivity increased across the experimental interventions, the increase was unrelated to changes in working conditions. Instead, workers may have increased their productivity in response to the experimenters' positive concerns about them and their working conditions (Roethlisberger, 1977) or to some combination of feedback about their output and financial reward (Parsons, 1974). Whatever the cause, the increased productivity was the result of variables that were unplanned and uncontrolled. Even survey research is an intervention that may result in unanticipated effects, including "reactivity as a method factor in assessment, the external validity of results, the motivation of the subjects to present a particular image, and the influence of the individual who administers the assessment device" (Kazdin, 1980, p. 257).

Unanticipated effects of research fall into three general categories (Warwick & Lininger, 1975). First, the researchers' goals and values may affect the intervention in unanticipated ways. Second, participants themselves or the community may make requests or demands that alter the research and its outcome. Finally, the funding source may, either symbolically or through overt action, be a source of pressure.

INTERVENTION EFFECTS OF RESEARCHER'S GOALS AND VALUES

The Hawthorne effect is one example of the researcher's assumptions influencing research outcome. Whether the outcome was due to increased morale because of experimenter attention or to the feedback of data and reward for performance, the researchers failed to anticipate the impact of their own behavior on the participants.

In community psychology, the goal of empowering participants has increased the practice of including participants in the research planning process. Although this practice does achieve the empowerment goal, it raises provocative methodological issues. For example, a colleague conducted a collaborative community project in which the community refused to include a control group in the research design. Only after the project was completed were participants able to understand the value of a control group. This researcher is left with the advantage of having trusted the community to make critical decisions about the research; it is assumed that she will be welcome to conduct future studies in that community. She is also left with disadvantages resulting from the scientific naiveté of the communal decision. She is not in a position to know whether the variables studied were in fact instrumental in bringing about the results. This uncertainty complicates both the planning of future programmatic research and the sharing of her work with professional colleagues through publication.

INTERVENTION EFFECTS OF COMMUNITY REQUESTS

Requests or demands from members of the community involved in the research can also have unanticipated effects. Two such unplanned requests complicated a program that was designed to assess the value of training human service workers to identify cases of child sexual abuse (Swift, 1986). First, although the research demonstrated the training to be successful, news of the project within the community generated numerous requests for services to child victims and their families—services that were essentially nonexistent at the time. Many of the human service workers participating in training were frequent targets of such requests. Their responses across the training period both benefited the research by providing case material and complicated it by resulting in participants gaining varying degrees of experience across the intervention period.

Second, a request came from participants who asked to meet with other professionals within the community who dealt with cases of child sexual abuse. The problem was that many were involved in the research as members of alternative experimental or control groups. Although their desire to form community teams was an excellent response to the community's needs, it created problems for the researcher. In retrospect, following Serrano-García's model (see Chapter 14 in this volume) of "horizontal" research planning with the community in more depth would have brought these issues to the surface earlier and smoothed research implementation.

INTERVENTION EFFECTS OF FUNDING SOURCE PRESSURE

One of the most troubling sources of pressure can be that generated by the research funding source. It is understandable that funders should specify research goals and objectives, and, in some cases, methodological practices as well. Major problems arise when the funding source is not neutral about outcome or when it challenges research that raises questions about its product or process. A familiar example is the tobacco industry, which takes the position that there is no connection between smoking and cancer despite the many studies that point to this connection.

A more subtle case of the influence of a funding source on research may arise from the image that it has in the community, rather than from any explicit position or demand it may make. A community psychologist and his research team, in seeking a sponsor for a smoking cessation program, considered a popular nationwide hamburger chain. The chain offered to underwrite the cost of distributing training literature. It carried high visibility and would have provided a constant, daily stream of families to receive the educational materials. The research team, in reflecting on the values projected by such a connection, considered the symbolism the chain represented—high salt, high caloric content, high fat—and decided the message conveyed was an inappropriate one to associate with their health-promotion research.

Colleagues have declined funding for research and education programs from the liquor industry and from certain popular national magazines because of concerns about both the freedom to design and report the research and the questionable image that such support could cast on the study.

In conclusion, in addition to the planned interventions implemented by experimenters, research can create unplanned and unanticipated interventions that may affect the research outcome or participants' lives. Three sources of such unanticipated interventions are the researcher's goals and values, requests from the community, and pressures from the funding source. The scientific community would benefit from increased attention to the issues raised by research as intervention.

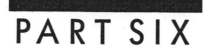

PART SIX

USING THEORY AND METHODS IN COMMUNITY RESEARCH

CHAPTER 16

REFLECTIONS ON A CONFERENCE
A. DARING TO BE DIFFERENT: A GRADUATE STUDENT'S PERSPECTIVE

CAROLYN L. FEIS

> The teacher who walks in the shadow of the temple, among his followers, gives not of his wisdom but rather of his faith and his lovingness. If he is indeed wise he does not bid you enter the house of his wisdom, but rather leads you to the threshold of your own mind.
>
> (Kahlil Gibran, *The Prophet,* p. 56)

There is no single correct solution to any social problem (Rappaport, 1981). In striving to be adventuresome in community psychology research, there is also no single correct method or theory. A psychological sense of community does not require that a community (including the discipline of community psychology) be homogeneous or conflict-free (Heller & Monahan, 1977).

Rappaport (1981) suggested that we must understand that there are many times when we will be pulled in two ways at once by two contrary notions. Because strain is a force that is neither positive nor negative (Heller & Monahan, 1977), these paradoxes should be a source of excitement for the field. For example, either research or action alone would be a disservice to the discipline (Kelly, 1984). A community psychologist is one who both acts and conceptualizes (Gatz & Liem, 1977), and each of these diverse goals should be encouraged (Patton, 1988). It is in the fusion of research and action that community psychology can best fulfill its dream.

Although community psychologists have a shared set of values, techniques, and theories, which act as the glue that holds us all together despite our diverse backgrounds and interests, it is necessary to remain open to any and all theories and methods that may help in each research endeavor. When developing research ideas, choosing methods, implementing research, reporting findings, and, most important, training graduate students, community psychologists must foster creativity and resist the temptation to fit all community psychologists into a single mold. My purpose here is to combine the interests of the discipline with the goals expressed in this book and translate them into recommendations for changes in graduate training and employment opportunities for young professionals that will promote innovative and adventuresome research.

Frequently, different research techniques, strategies, or methodologies are discussed as categories that are mutually exclusive. This form of dichotomous thinking, however, is inappropriate in community psychology. These strategies should be seen as a rich pool from which we may select the method that is most appropriate for the tasks at hand. The unique contributions of each technique may be preserved so that the use of one does not diminish the merits of another. Combining strategies can contribute to the field in ways that produce a total result that may be greater than the sum of its parts. The best chance of finding solutions to social problems is when multiple approaches are used so that the strengths of each compensate for the weaknesses of the others (Shadish, Cook, & Houts, 1986).

The problem-orientation of community psychology encourages and promotes the use of theories and methods from other areas of psychology and from disciplines outside of psychology. Although there are concepts from these disciplines that are important to community psychology, we must not become subordinate to any one discipline (Fairweather, 1980). One's identity as a community psychologist should be separate from one's association with another field of study.

Social problems do not respect disciplinary boundaries (Sandler & Keller, 1984), and, as a result, answers to social problems cannot be found within a single academic discipline. It is not that these other theories are bad for the profession; rather, it is that they do not define community psychology. The existence of clinical-community, organizational-community, developmental-community psychologists, and so on illustrates that these other disciplines remain separate and distinct from that which is community psychology. It is not—and *should not* be—the obligation or responsibility of community psychology to teach the theories of other disciplines. However, community psychology training programs must provide students with the opportunity to learn them.

Just as diversity in both theory and methodology is promoted as a strength of community psychology, so should it be cultivated in the graduate training of community psychologists. Rappaport (1977) has argued that the content of traditional psychology must supplement, not dominate, the training of future com-

This chapter and my ideas have been enriched by many discussions with Kelly Hazel and Nancy Burgoyne. Their contributions are invaluable and go beyond any specific citation.

munity psychologists. The old paradigms have failed to address social problems adequately, and if community psychology does not allow students the freedom to try new methods and research techniques and to explore new paradigms, it will also fail.

Diversity, creativity, and *flexibility* should be the key words in graduate training. Trickett (1984) has argued that training programs should be seen as a greenhouse for developing the values, issues, and intervention demands of the field. Furthermore, Hazel (1988) argued that graduate training should allow students to search for new, innovative ideas that break the rules and may even seem impractical. Creativity is the foundation on which risk-taking is built.

Graduate students in community psychology are, by definition, risk-takers, who are willing to try something new because it is the right thing to do (Fairweather, 1980). It is incumbent of graduate training programs to help students become intelligent risk-takers. Graduate trainers and employers of new students need to educate their students by encouraging them to learn all that they can without letting this knowledge restrict or stifle their development of ideas or choice of methods. Graduate training should be viewed, like any other social problem, as having multiple approaches and solutions and should be presented in ways that encourage and develop students' passion. Graduate training should empower students, where *empowerment* is defined by the number of choices one *feels* he or she has and by knowing these choices, using them, and being successful at them. This may require changes in existing graduate curricula. Because change is rooted in action, I offer these suggestions for change.

1. *Weave the idea of adventuresome research into the entire graduate curriculum.* In methods courses, this may involve adding a sense of reality, such as evaluating research in terms of how it was or was not adventuresome and brainstorming about how it might have been so. It may also mean developing courses that are entirely experiential in nature. Practicum courses do not require traditional readings. Instead, field trips or guest speakers should be used to expose students, firsthand, to the realities of the field. Coursework can be expanded beyond the traditional literature, and alternative sources in which social problems have been dramatized in both fictional and nonfictional accounts can be examined.

2. *Encourage true collaboration.* Although this may involve working with people in traditional areas of psychology, it also means collaborating with individuals from other disciplines and with community members. Such efforts may require changes at the departmental level, such as eliminating degree requirements that restrict opportunities for collaboration or even adding ones that encourage it. Encouraging students to become involved in nontraditional practicum settings instead of or, if necessary, in addition to sites approved by the American Psychological Association, should also occur. More of the ideas of community psychology should be brought into clinical-community psychology programs, so that the "community" half no longer takes a back seat to the "clinical" half.

3. *Involve students.* Most faculty members seek and obtain outside funding

to conduct research projects that often involve students. Students should be included in the original conceptualization of these projects rather than handed a product to implement. First, students will bring to the process unique perspectives, which may improve the quality of the research and increase both the efficacy and relevance of the project. Second, and more important for the students, they will learn, firsthand, how the research process unfolds, how to develop ideas, and how to work cooperatively in doing so.

4. *Respect the contributions that students can make.* One of the "minitheories" of community psychology is that the community should be involved in decision making in problem definition and in implementation of interventions. Within the context of a graduate training program, this means that students should be involved in decisions that affect their training experience, such as issues of curriculum, practicum, committee membership, and so on. Training programs should be participatory democracies. Training should not be done *to* students, but, rather *with* students.

5. *Support students.* As reviewers of thesis and dissertation proposals, it is important that faculty members recognize ideas that may fall short in some areas but excel in the areas toward which the field is trying to move. For example, what a research proposal lacks in rigor, it may make up for in relevance. As adventuresome research becomes more important to the field, it may be necessary to shift the focus to those areas in which research proposals are attempting to break new ground.

Although these five changes are necessary to empower students and promote adventuresome research, they are not sufficient. It is also necessary to reassure students that the consequences of truly adventuresome research will not restrict their employment opportunities. This requires a commitment from employers to accept innovation in graduate training. First, employers must look beyond the number of publications on a vita. Research that is longitudinal, involves implementing interventions in a community organization, or is not part of a faculty member's ongoing research project will take longer to complete and may result in fewer publications. Furthermore, it is necessary to acknowledge publications not found in refereed academic journals. A substantial portion of policy-related publications are produced as internal or technical reports that are used to create change within an organization. This is the action side of adventuresome research, and it should be recognized for the unique contribution that it can make to community psychology. Finally, employers must look beyond publications. It is important to recognize the value of research and work experiences outside of the university. Students who have searched beyond the university for mentors should not be judged more harshly than those who have found them within the university. Furthermore, the experience that is gained by working outside the university should be appreciated. The community, as a training site, should be viewed as a resource not only for the student, but also for what that student brings back to the academic department.

In order to truly foster adventuresome research in graduate training, it is necessary for faculty to be creative in their thinking about their students' ideas, to lead by doing, and to show their mistakes to their students so that all may learn from them. Nothing magical happens on the day that a doctorate degree is earned that makes someone interested in or able to conduct adventuresome research. This interest and ability must come from a combination of the passion inside of the student and the training experiences that have developed and expanded his or her talents and interests.

B. A CAUTIONARY NOTE ABOUT ADVENTURESOME RESEARCH: MUSINGS OF A JUNIOR RESEARCHER

ANA MARI CAUCE

This volume focuses on our scientific research and how it informs us about our world and our attempts to change it. However, research is not solely the path that we follow in our pursuit of knowledge-seeking. It is also one of our best avenues for legitimizing knowledge. Despite the shortcomings of research, "neither God nor tradition is privileged with the same credibility as scientific rationality in modern cultures" (Harding, 1986). Therefore, discussion of the theories and methods that guide our research is of extreme importance. Such discussions have implications not only for how we go about our individual scholarly business, but also for how we train our student-colleagues and present our work to the public.

It is because of this that I am dismayed by what appears to be a trend toward the summary dismissal of all things associated with a positivist tradition and an all-too-eager embrace of so-called "adventuresome" research. The tone of the discussions at the conference associated with this volume cannot be fully captured here, but suffice it to say that one conference participant described it as "logical positivism bashing," and I believe that was an apt description.

Extreme positivist perspectives are easy targets for attacks. The doctrine of logical positivism, as elaborated by the Vienna Circle and operationalized within psychology by early radical behaviorist programs, purports to define the correct methods and type of problems to be pursued through rational scientific inquiry, which was viewed as the *only* method that could lead us to proper truths. Not only is this naively inductivist position an affront to myriad forms of knowing, including most scholarship within the arts and humanities, but it is also flawed in terms of its own logic. For example, in the mid-18th century, Hume had already noted that the basic underpinnings of the inductivist method could not be supported by induction itself (cf. Russell, 1945).

Extreme positivist perspectives are not only narrow and faulty in their logic, but they also reify the commonly held myth of the scientist as a neutral and objective observer. As a Hispanic woman and a feminist, I am well aware of how such erroneous beliefs have helped to maintain and to legitimize—in part through science—a society that is far from neutral in its characterizations and treatment of women and people of color. In the 1930s and 1940s, Karl Popper was eloquently and incisively pointing out the inextricable commingling of theory and observation.[1] He stated that scientific enterprises did not begin with neutral observations that then proceeded to inductive generalization and hypothesis testing, experimentation, verification, and, in the end, produced knowledge or truth. Instead, he argued that the scientist begins by posing a problem, already couched in theory-driven terms, which is then followed by observation, experimentation, possible refutation, and, finally, ends with a justification for a *preferred* theory. (For a fuller elaboration of Popper's arguments see Chalmers, 1976, or Magee, 1973.)

Therefore, at this time, I fear that, in so singularly attacking logical positivism, we have created a straw man for empiricism more generally and for attempts at precise measurement and the study of "real-world" problems in the laboratory more specifically. Furthermore, I am concerned that, in our attempts to replace what we describe as a pervasive paradigm in psychology, we are incorrectly characterizing the nature of our field and glossing over the problematic sociological, as opposed to epistemological, context within which community psychology research is produced.

As the excellent expositions, of behavioral, developmental, organizational, empowerment, and ecological theory in this volume so aptly illustrate, we are undoubtedly a multiperspective discipline. Methodological approaches that highlight experimental control and rigor may enjoy more academically prestigious venues for publication. Yet multiple methodological approaches are also evident in our scientific endeavors. Community psychology's most renowned and respected contributors, both past and present, have not been traditional researchers working from a narrow positivist framework. We are not now, nor have we ever been, constricted by any one paradigm, as has been more the case in the physical and natural sciences. If, as some imply, our field is losing its vibrancy and moral convictions or passion, it is surely not because we are operating in some positivist stranglehold. As a field, we are not lacking creative ideas or complex, contextually sensitive insights gleaned from value-driven and politicized inquiry.[2] Indeed, as a junior researcher, I often believe that what is most lacking are exemplars of

---

[1]One could replace the word *theory* with the word *values* and the argument would remain essentially unchanged.

[2]The work of community psychologists such as Sarason, Albee, many of the contributors to this volume, and countless others stands as examples of this.

the "how tos" of bringing more empirical research practices in line with the values and perspectives extolled. In this vein, I urge the senior researcher in our field to be less rhetorical in their exhortations toward adventure and to lead us, instead, by example.

An interplay between controlled, careful, and precise experimental methods and quasi-experimental, qualitative, and less intrusive approaches is not only desirable—it is essential to advancing our knowledge about community phenomena. Just as there is no specific theory that is in all cases more desirable, morally superior, or a "best expression" of our research questions, so I believe the same is true of methods.

We should, however, acknowledge that there *are* inherent tensions between the desire for precision and parsimony and the need to be ecologically and contextually sensitive. It may be a truism that we do not have to sacrifice precision for ecological validity, but, in practice, this often happens. Our ethical standards, which should acknowledge that truly horizontal relationships in research are not only often impossible to establish but also extremely difficult to maintain, prevent us from exercising the same levels of experimental control in real-world settings as might be possible in laboratory or analogue studies. Even when dealing with survey research, for example, I think that in many instances it is wasteful of community resources *not* to begin the process of questionnaire construction and validation with college students. Then, when we work with community participants, we can circumvent some of the problems inherent in the hit-and-miss nature of such projects.

My own collaborative work with programs in the community has led me to question the extent to which we, the academic researchers in our field, have embraced the principles of horizontal research relationships and action-oriented research. Indeed, I have been impressed by the number of small, high-quality, preventively oriented programs already quietly operating in our local communities and schools. In contrast to those that I associate with community psychologists, such programs are smaller in scale, are less theoretically articulated, and are run by the "Mrs. Dewars of the world.[3] They are also locally rooted, have emerged from the community with a full awareness of its standards and values, and provide good services. It is my emergent knowledge about prevention and my personal and professional values (shaped, in part, by the rhetoric of community psychology) that have led such programs to welcome my collaboration. But it is my training in empirical research design and quantitative methods that they most appreciate and value. When it comes to structuring and delivering services, the program developers and staff are clearly the experts, although I have at times offered suggestions. When it comes to designing the research, my student-colleagues and I are the experts, although program staff, and at times participants, are involved in every step of decision making. Our mutual desire to create a

---

[3]See Sarason, Carroll, Maton, Cohen, and Lorentz (1977) for a description of the original "Mrs. Dewar."

climate for such endeavors that is enriching, and perhaps empowering, for all concerned does not allow us to conduct what, from a purely positivist standpoint, would be considered the best science. Nonetheless, I believe such collaborations are best characterized as balanced, not horizontal. In considering them fully horizontal, I would be shirking the responsibilities that go along with the prestige and status that society accords to me as a university-based scientist.[4]

In addition to working with these programs to develop better methods of evaluation, I think the best way that I can serve them is by continuing to develop my research program in ways that provide links between the outcomes that they can most readily measure and the outcomes that are most convincing to funding agencies and the public. For example, I have been working with a community-based parenting program for low-socioeconomic-status teenage mothers. Limited funds for evaluation and the decision to be minimally intrusive into the lives of participants make it unlikely that we can link program participation to better parent-child relationships. Yet we should be able to show that participant mothers report higher levels of self-esteem, less social isolation, and stronger social support networks at the program's end. The nascent, sometimes laboratory-based, research literature linking mothers' higher social support levels to warmer family environments and more desirable parent-child interactions, although not what many would call adventuresome, can be used to help such programs survive in a conservative fiscal environment.

My own graduate and undergraduate student colleagues, most of whom are ethnic minority women, are less afraid to be adventuresome than I, and they bring immense passion to their work. Yet I feel it my responsibility, as their mentor, to ensure that they spend as much time in the somewhat anachronistic atmosphere of the academy, poring over thick tomes of research design and computer printouts, as they do in the community. Moreover, I often remind them that what defines intelligent risk-taking (which goes hand-in-hand with adventure-some approaches) depends largely on one's position in the academic and social hierarchy.

Lest we become enamored of our own rhetoric about moving away from a psychology preoccupied with white rats and White college students, let us remember that such preoccupations are not unrelated to the fact that we have been, and continue to be, a community of primarily White researchers. Moreover, I cannot help but be skeptical about the diversity of observations, insights, and research relationships possible as long as this is so, regardless of what epistemologies are in vogue. The fact that we expound upon epistemologies that highlight the values and personal characteristics of the researcher while giving considerably less emphasis to the sociological makeup of our researcher community (and how it contrasts to the researched community) does little to quell such skepticism.

The possibility of transforming our research enterprises in ways that are more humane, ecologically valid, and empowering is exciting. I would urge more

---

[4]This is the case whether or not such status and prestige is rightfully accorded.

caution and humility, however, in the face of the enormous challenges before us. It may be time to ask ourselves a series of questions posed by Donna Haraway, a historian of science (quoted in Harding, 1986). I have paraphrased these questions by substituting the term *community* where she had used the word *feminist*:

> Is there a specifically community theory of knowledge which is analogous in its implications to theories which are the heritage of Greek science and of the scientific revolution of the seventeenth century? Would a community epistemology informing scientific inquiry be a family member to existing theories of representation and philosophical realism? Or should community psychologists adopt a radical form of epistemology that denies the possibility of access to a real world and objective standpoint? Would community standards of knowledge genuinely end the dilemma of the cleavage between subject and object or between noninvasive knowing and prediction and control? Does community psychology offer insight into the connections between science and humanism? Do community psychologists have anything new to say about the vexed relations of knowledge and power? Would community authority and power to name give the world a new identity, a new story?

This self-analysis is too much to expect from our young field, but is not too much to ask. Working with our fullest diversity of theories, research methods, and researchers, we may someday come closer to answering the final set of questions by saying *Yes*.

C. PARTIAL PARADIGMS AND PROFESSIONAL IDENTITY: OBSERVATIONS ON THE STATE OF COMMUNITY PSYCHOLOGY RESEARCH

EDISON J. TRICKETT

Attending the exciting conference that led to this book, I was frequently reminded of Lily Tomlin's comment in her one-person show, "The Search for Signs of Intelligent Life in the Universe." At one point she says, "All my life I've always wanted to *be* somebody. But I see now I should have been more specific" (Wagner, p. 35). She continues: "It's not that I lack ambition. I *am* ambitious in the sense that I want to be more than I am now. But if I were truly ambitious, I think I'd already be more than I am now" (p. 35).

The wide-ranging agenda of this volume and its preceding conference, undergirded by the theme of adventuresome research, reflects both the historically broad ambition of community psychology—the wanting to "be somebody"—and its continuing diffuse character—"I see now I should have been more specific."

It also highlights the underlying concern that progress in the field has not yet fulfilled the aspirations surrounding the field's origins. The call for adventuresome research is partially fueled by the worry that if community psychology were truly ambitious—in its carings, risks, and paradigms—it would already be more than it is now. The existence of the September 1988 Chicago conference challenges us to create research as adventuresome as the values of the field itself. A special challenge confronts senior scholars in the field: to avoid the seductions of success at the expense of the evolution of the field. The following comments reflect my understanding of the dual themes of ambition and diffusion in community psychology research. A number of potential "next steps" for the evolution of the field's research paradigms come from this understanding.

PARTIAL PARADIGM ACQUISITION: ACHIEVING CONGRUENCE BETWEEN VALUES AND RESEARCH

Historical Values and Themes

In creating a context for adventuresome research in community psychology, it is useful to review some of the field's initial guiding assumptions and how, in terms of our research behavior, they have played out over time. Let me mention three themes and a general perspective embodying those themes that surfaced at the Swampscott conference (Bennett et al., 1966). The themes involve levels of analysis of behavior, a commitment to poor and minority populations, and collaboration between scientist and citizen. The general perspective embodying these themes for me is an ecological approach to research and intervention.

Each of the three themes reflects community psychology's disagreement with the dominant psychological paradigms at the time of its creation. With respect to the level of analysis of behavior, our new field asserted the importance of understanding how the social context and social processes affect behavior and development. The research agenda of this theme focuses on the assessment of social systems and the interdependence of individuals and those social systems. The critique behind this initiative toward contextualizing behavior lies in psychology's emphasis on conducting research on individuals, with a relative disregard for history and context (see Sarason, 1981). The theme of commitment to poor and minority populations emphasized community psychology's value stance toward the disempowered. The research critique behind this commitment included the need to develop nonlaboratory methodologies, to expand the participants in research beyond college students, and to deal conceptually with the issue of the ecological validity of research data. The theme of collaboration was intended to create a redefinition of the relationship between citizen and scientist. Here, the values centered on creating horizontal collaboration rather than hierarchical rela-

---

I wish to thank Dr. Kathleen D. Schmid for her helpful comments on these remarks.

tionships—the notion of differential expertise rather than the imagery of doctor and patient.

Underlying these three themes was a general belief in the value of an ecological perspective on behavior and an active "participant-conceptualizer"[1] research role for the community psychologist. Such a perspective would be one that would unravel the impact of differing levels of analysis of social systems on individual and group behavior, that would contextualize individual behavior in a sociocultural matrix, and that would incorporate collaboration with citizens in defining and carrying out the research enterprise (see Bennett et al., 1966).

Upon rereading the proceedings of the Swampscott conference (Bennett et al., 1966), it seems clear that the vision of and hopes for community psychology triumphed over specific ideas about how to translate these values into action. Thus, although providing a potentially visionary framework for the creation of a new field based on alternative assumptions about behavior, social values, and research relationships, the Swampscott conference left the task of paradigmatic elaboration to subsequent generations of community psychologists. This elaboration, although constantly progressing, has not come easily.

Persuasion and Conversion as Stages in Paradigm Elaboration

Reviews of published literature in community psychology suggest that the field is still working out the paradigm elaborations of its origins in the search for a distinctive identity that is based on distinctive perspectives. Previously published analyses suggest that the research literature in the field does not yet predominantly reflect the three themes discussed earlier. Thus, Novaco and Monahan (1980) and McClure et al. (1980) agree that, if the focus of community psychology is on institutional change and ecological analysis, most of the published work in the field does not reflect this premise. Instead, the level of analysis remains predominantly at the individual level. Similar analyses by Loo, Fong, and Iwamasa (1988) and by Walsh (1987b) reach comparable conclusions about lack of emphasis on minority populations and descriptions of collaborative research relationships. To be sure, there are examples that counteract the dominant body of work in the field (e.g., Kelly & Hess, 1987; Seidman, 1983; Trickett & Birman, 1987).

Kuhn (1970), in *The Structure of Scientific Revolutions*, presents one perspective on the development of new paradigms that casts community psychology's confrontations with its premises in a useful light. He asserts that debates about paradigms are debates about premises that, because they are fundamental and often unconscious, are very difficult to unravel and explicate fully. Thus, some surface beliefs may be altered without the belief-holder internalizing the implications for the more fundamental premises.

---

[1]Credit for this increasingly apt phrase goes to Dr. Forrest Tyler, a participant-conceptualizer at the Swampscott conference.

In the process of adopting new paradigms, Kuhn (1970) distinguishes between persuasion and conversion. *Persuasion* implies an intellectual choice to develop the implications of new premises. Such a choice, however, is not necessarily sufficient for *conversion* to the paradigm.

> To translate a theory or worldview into one's own language is not to make it one's own. For that, one must go native, discover that one is thinking in and working in, not merely translating out of, a language that was previously foreign . . . one may be fully persuaded of the new view but . . . unable to internalize it and be at home with the world it helps to shape. (p. 204)

Persuasion, although potentially on the road to conversion, requires an ongoing monitoring and introspection about the implications of paradigm assumptions if it is to result in conversion or the internalization of a new worldview. This volume represents a timely forum for furthering the implications of various paradigms still emerging in our field. In highlighting five different perspectives, community psychology is simultaneously acknowledging a potentially healthy set of additive ideas and a potentially confusing set of diffuse options for the future.

The goal of adventuresome research rests on the elaboration of these varied perspectives and their contributions to the subject matter of community psychology. Thus, one criterion for adventuresome research in community psychology involves research that is explicitly paradigmatic. Although no research is paradigm-free, research does differ in the degree to which it explicitly attempts to stretch and elaborate on paradigm assumptions. Such research is both theory driven and assumptions-underlying-the-theory driven. Much of the prototype for this kind of work is evolving in other areas of inquiry that, like community psychology, have begun as critiques of dominant perspectives. Thus, Harding (1987) provided a feminist perspective on philosophy of science that carries pervasive implications for how to reconceptualize research questions and the research process as it involves issues of gender. In like manner, Jones (1986) and Ramirez (1983) have generated frameworks for reconceptualizing research involving culturally diverse populations. The ongoing need is conceptual: To deepen the awareness of the implications of our underlying paradigm assumptions. This will, in turn, lead to a set of community psychologies that can, only then, provide the bases for a distinctive field.

A second criterion for adventuresome research involves a commitment to more explicit interchange and mutual criticism about our varied perspectives. In our efforts to promote innovation and the development of new ways of thinking, we have been rightly supportive of the value of supporting diversity within the field in terms of research questions, perspectives, and activities. What is now needed is a more focused "between perspective" discussion to develop the complementarities and disparities in varied points of view. Respectful mutual criticism can deepen our paradigmatic understanding.

ECOLOGY AS A METAPHOR FOR COMMUNITY PSYCHOLOGY

As previously mentioned, the general notion of *ecology* as one perspective for community psychology has existed since the Swampscott conference. The current volume affirms the centrality of contextual understandings of people, policies, and programs as an overarching theme for the field. The chapters in this volume highlight both the promise and the problems in acquiring such an ecological perspective. The concept of empowerment, for example, is potentially mischievous if not embedded in the specific goals, values, processes, and definitions of power that have local relevance. Unless grounded in local conditions, empowerment efforts could become another exercise in psychological imperialism or the imposing of external and potentially alien ideology. The notion of collaboration is also necessarily linked to the context and phenomenology of those with whom we wish to collaborate. And the occurrence of suggestions about adding contextual descriptions in articles published in community journals further suggests that ecological leanings are on the rise.

Indeed, the metaphor of ecology has been initially used to explicate the three Swampscott conference themes previously mentioned (e.g., Bronfenbrenner, 1979; Kelly, 1986; Trickett, 1984). Still, the acquisition of an ecological perspective within community psychology is in need of considerable elaboration.

With respect to publication practices, for example, Hobfoll remarked during the September 1988 conference that "our discussion of ecology usually happens in the discussion section," where post hoc explanation compensates for a lack of initial framing of research questions that derive from an ecological framework. Adding richness to the description of the contexts where the research occurs and discussing the relationships between researcher and citizen were also suggested as ways of increasing the ecological flavor of research reports. Although providing useful "baby steps" toward an ecological understanding of phenomena, such efforts represent steps toward persuasion, not conversion. Rather, truly adventuresome ecological research would integrate the research relationship with the scope, quality, and impact of the data, it would assess interventions across settings and levels of analysis; and it would develop constructs that derive their power from a collaborative research process.

Of particular concern in this regard has been the relative lack of emphasis—in this column and in the field—on the articulation of cultural diversity as a substantive (in addition to political) aspect of community psychology theory and research. An ecologically oriented community psychology affirms the positive values of cultural diversity; it explicitly acknowledges the sociocultural embeddedness of individuals whose lives are influenced by events occurring at multiple levels of analysis; it affirms that opportunities are not randomly distributed across race and gender and that social structures are not equally supportive for minorities, women, gays and lesbians, and those with disabilities. By focusing on the relationship of culturally diverse individuals whose multiple group identifications interact in varying ways with the mediating structures of the broader culture, an ecological metaphor can provide a contextual grounding for the empowerment and prevention efforts of the field.

An ecological perspective may also be of use to the American Psychological Association's Division of Community Psychology as it attempts to promote issues of human diversity within its own membership and activities. Approaching varied constituencies from a perspective that acknowledges their distinctive cultural positions will allow a clearer understanding of how policies, practices, and rituals of the division may be differently viewed by different constituencies. Success in this area will simultaneously increase the quality and quantity of resources to further the goals of the division and the field.

In summary, then, adventuresome research is related to the articulation and elaboration of paradigms that promote the distinctive professional identity of community psychology. I am suggesting that the overarching concept of ecology be pursued as one salient, unifying metaphor. This pursuit involves issues of epistemology, concepts, and a continual vigilance in order to understand how individuals and the social context interact. Such work requires time; it entails varying kinds of risks because of its non-normative nature; it requires generating networks of support and developing resources to sustain those networks. Where risks are to be taken, the primary responsibility lies with those of us who can best afford to take them. Senior researchers have a special responsibility to model and to nurture the kinds of research problems and research relationships that the field nominates as its "adventures."

D. WHAT CAN WE LEARN ABOUT PROBLEMS IN COMMUNITY RESEARCH BY COMPARING IT WITH PROGRAM EVALUATION?

WILLIAM R. SHADISH, JR.

In Chapter 2, I described a logic and some criteria for judging the merits of community research. I hoped that these prescriptions might reach out to challenge community researchers without seeming too directly confronting. Yet the subsequent chapters lead me to think that the abstractness of that logic and those criteria may have discouraged their concrete application. Hence, I would like to be more concrete in these closing comments, using the logic and the criteria to explore some problems with community research. Of course, many community researchers are doing good research by these standards, and they represent exceptions to the criticisms that follow. However, I do think that they are the exceptions and not the rule, so that the following criticisms are broadly true. I hope these remarks will open a constructive dialogue about the strengths and weaknesses of a field that I admire greatly.

To aid in my task, I would like to compare community psychology with program evaluation, for both logical and pragmatic reasons. As noted in Chapter 2, the second step of the logic of valuing is standard-setting, and the most practical standard is usually comparative—how the thing being evaluated is faring under one approach in comparison with another approach to achieve the same ends. To the degree that the two fields share social problem solving as a goal, their activities and accomplishments serve as comparative standards for each other. My subsequent comments criticize the merits of community research more than those of program evaluation only because community research is the topic of this book. Program evaluation can be soundly criticized, too, and I have done so myself on many occasions.

Pragmatically, the comparison is justified because the two fields share common historical roots. Both blossomed in the social reform fervor of the 1960s, and both had similar roots in psychology's experimental tradition. The two specialties operate under different social structures, however—a situation that I think has profound implications for how the fields function. Community psychology developed primarily as an academic specialty with a social structure typical of that setting. Like most academic specialties, the specifics of community research are created by faculty members who pursue research programs that are driven more by personal curiosities and values than by externally imposed demands. There is nothing in the structure of academia that requires particular attention to social problem solving.

Granted, some community psychologists pursue highly problem-oriented research—(e.g., Geller's work on seat belts and Winett and colleagues' on energy conservation), but I suspect that such instances occur because of a coincidental isomorphism between social problems and personal interests (in both the psychological and material sense), not because the specialty places any selective value on such achievements. By contrast, program evaluation developed as a profession that is based largely in social structures associated with addressing social problems. Its structure is intimately interwoven with social policy structures from which researchers cannot withdraw without withdrawing, to a large degree, from the profession itself. In ways that academically based specialties have not, program evaluation has had to respond to demands to show how it is useful in social problem solving, to cope with the diversity of values that drive the political

That this portion of the chapter is in any way more cogent or civilized than in its original form is largely due to the thoughtful and patient criticisms of a host of community researchers and other colleagues, including the following: Tom Cook, Fern Chertok, Lenny Jason, Chris Keys, Stephanie Riger, Ed Seidman, Beth Shinn, and Pat Tolan. Of course, I will continue to take full responsibility for all the mistakes still present.

process, and to integrate methodological and epistemological perspectives from the many diverse disciplines that routinely compete for evaluative dollars. Consequently, it has been more responsive to these external demands and has developed theories of research that are better tailored to cope with them. In our 1986 *Annual Review of Psychology* chapter, Cook and I called program evaluation "the worldly science" partly for these reasons—it is intimately and necessarily immersed in the world so that there is no hiding from the harsh lessons about social problem solving. Thus, although it is like community psychology in many ways, its different social structure has curtailed the academic insularity that I think still characterizes community psychology.

In the context of this comparison, then, the first observation is that a fundamental assumption of my argument may be wrong. Specifically, the decisions that drive the exact form of community research—for example, what questions to ask, what interventions to study, or how to study them—seem to have less to do with trying to solve social problems than they do with maintaining a sense of "community identity." This community identity apparently requires that research have certain values (e.g., working with the disenfranchised), rest on certain concepts (e.g., deinstitutionalization, ecology, a psychological sense of community), and focus on certain levels of intervention (e.g., in local communities), regardless of whether they are the best or the only means of tackling a particular social problem These requirements lead to an interesting dilemma. Suppose I make a useful contribution to social problem solving, yet I do so at, say, the state or federal rather than the community level or by pursuing values that are not consonant with the majority of community researchers (both things are true in my work on long-term care for the mentally ill, where one of my goals has been to encourage better federal and state policies regarding institutionalization). I will apparently be perceived as not engaging in good community research. That says something about what community psychology hopes to accomplish. It is willing to sacrifice some important routes to social problem solving in order to maintain a sense of community identity. It is not obvious why, so that the matter deserves extended debate.

Second, relative to program evaluation, which has always been an extremely disputatious field, I am struck by the lack of extensive, comparative, mutual criticism among community researchers. For example, the five theoretical presentations following my opening chapter have each done an admirable job of presenting the strengths of the perspectives. Understandably, many community researchers will be tempted to adopt one of these perspectives in their work— presumably the best one. But which is best? Presumably the one with, roughly speaking, the most strengths and the fewest weaknesses on some set of criteria for good community research. However, except for Fawcett's presentation of the behavior-analytic model (Chapter 7), there is little discussion about what each approach cannot do, either on its own terms or in comparison with the other four competitors. To the extent that any such comparisons are done, they are usually made with some abstract "traditional research paradigm" that may be more straw man than reality. Thus, after reading the five approaches, the reader is left with a good sense of the internal strengths of each approach as judged on its own terms, but with little sense of its strengths relative to the others and almost no sense of its weaknesses. Remedying such omissions requires both self-criticism and collegial criticism, so that community researchers can know when, where, and why to adopt part or all of each approach. I am told that, for many reasons, community psychology has had an unwritten norm against extensive mutual criticisms. An unfortunate side effect of this norm is that the general lack of discussion of such matters leaves the field with little sense of its limits.

This ill-formed sense of limits is fostered even more to the extent that community research is not criticized from those outside the field, which would help us to discover constant sources of bias across all approaches to community research. For example, to the extent that all approaches recommend working with the disadvantaged, community research as a whole incurs some limits that I will discuss further in a moment. In some sense, this comparison of community research to program evaluation is intended as just such an enlightening exercise—a chance to see ourselves from a new perspective that might help us to recognize and, if we want, transcend any paradigmatic myopias that we have developed in community research as a whole.

Third, relative to program evaluation, community research seems to devote less attention to discussing the four issues that gave rise to the criteria of merit that I nominated in Chapter 2 as important in judging the merits of community research. This may, of course, be a function of different researchers having different visions of the field. The issues that *I* think are most important are closely tied to my notions about social problem solving and would be of less relevance to those with different goals. Whatever the reason, however, it is not clear how often most community researchers think about these issues. I noted that there are rarely "correct" answers to these four key issues, but that, instead, there are options and trade-offs, each with different advantages and disadvantages. Under this conceptualization, the key is to avoid any constant biases across community research as a whole, whereby options with the same advantages and disadvantages come to dominate and other options that might yield very different perspectives are mostly overlooked. It is this matter of constant biases in response to the four issues that leads to my concern.

One such problem may be a constant bias concerning values. Admirably, community research has encouraged the clear and explicit acknowledgment of its values, reflected in phrases and words that signal those commitments: working with the disenfranchised, advocacy, horizontal relationships, empowerment, collaborative research relationships. Each of these concepts, by itself, can be a good idea, of course, and can have subtly important implications for community research. But this explicitness about values may not have been accompanied by an equally thoughtful consideration of value pluralism. It seems to me that, across community psychology as a whole, the values in the field disproportionately represent the left side of the political spectrum, with an almost hostile rejection of alternative value systems, particularly toward those from the right side of the spectrum. There seems to be less of a sense of the pluralism of values that drives interest-group democracy in the United States, of how self-defeating it can be to champion a narrow set of prescriptive values, and of how helpful it can be to deliberately represent a broad range of values (descriptive values) bearing on an issue in one's research (including one's own values, of course). Many community researchers seem to find it abhorrent to include in their research values that they do not personally share, partly because of the distaste that they feel for some values, and partly because they fear that by representing those values they will somehow foster them. The latter objection is, in fact, a risk of descriptive valuing, because the data sometimes support our opponents' position more than our own. That is the nature of data-based research. It does not always tell us what we want to hear. To be sure, we will never allow data to constitute the sole arbiter of our social and political actions, and there are good reasons to act against certain values even in the face of contradictory data. But one would have to have an almost frightening sense of omniscience to think that one can enter the political arena and not encounter well-reasoned and data-based arguments that support values that differ from one's own. Community researchers should represent an array of values in their work if for no other reason than to anticipate and counter such arguments effectively. In the process, I think they will discover how useful the descriptive valuing approach can be. Through it, we often encounter legitimate alternatives that expand our inevitably egocentric worldview, and, in turn, we develop the reputation of trusted advisers who can provide a broad perspective about the pros and cons of the issue of the day.

Next, consider some possible problems with the implicit theories of social problem solving and social change in community research. First, there seems to be little attention paid to the question of what should count as an important problem, so that poverty and social support are discussed as if they were equally important. If we prioritized a list of problems, however, would social support really be so high on that list as to deserve the extensive attention that it now receives in the community research literature? Possibly not, because a whole host of other problems may have more plausible and widespread links to harms done, to dollars lost, to other important problems to which they are interconnected, and to currently salient policy issues. Where are we getting our problem agenda from? From academic interests? From things that are convenient to study? Should we be thinking about alternative agendas?

Second, with a few exceptions, when they address these problems, community researchers tend to think small rather than big in the interventions that they study, and they tend to avoid state and federal policy research. Of course, these interventions are not small from the perspective of a field that developed community interventions that are considerably bigger than the individual clinical interventions that were almost completely dominant in psychology 20 years ago. But a "no holds barred" approach to social problem solving must not exclude any reasonable levels of intervention, and the policy level with its attendant large-scale social programs can be a powerful avenue. We have yet to explore it as much as we could.

Third, the heritage of the "experimenting society" is still an unduly strong undercurrent in community research. Experimenting with local innovations does give a sense of the possible and can help us to evaluate the radical options that a fundamentally conservative social system might otherwise overlook. We need such research to test limits and to provide a grab bag of options into which we can reach when the rare opportunities for major change present themselves. However, I would like to see more balanced consideration of whether one's favorite local intervention is feasible as a widespread solution to a problem, recognition of the fundamentally conservative nature of change in society, and attention to a more incrementalist approach to change. Sometimes we should be willing to sacrifice novelty for implementability.

I would also like to see community researchers give more thought to how they expect their research to be useful. The field still seems to be greatly influenced by its academic heritage, in which publishing is the main vehicle to facilitate use, in which academic colleagues are the main intended users, and in which a retreat to the ivory tower allows one to avoid serious consideration of the issue. All this leads to the erroneous notion that we can do nothing to understand the possible future impacts and benefits of present research. In program evaluation, one of the major failures of early approaches like "the experimenting society" was the perception that they failed to produce research that was used. For example, hopes that successfully evaluated innovations would be adopted when those results were disseminated were quickly dashed. It turned out that most of this kind of information is used more for "tinkering at the margins" than for disseminating and adopting demonstration projects wholesale. This fact led program evaluators to search widely for alternative research models that might produce more useful results for that tinkering—sometimes inventing their own methods, as with Wholey's "evaluability assessment" and "sequential purchase of information," and sometimes borrowing from other specialties with more experience in policy and decision making, as with Weiss's (Weiss & Bucuvalas, 1980) discussion of factors facilitating the conceptual use of research. Today, program evaluation uses an eclectic set of techniques to produce results that may be useful in different ways, depending on the kind and level of change desired and on the demands under which the researcher operates. I would like to see those technologies and theories about use disseminated more to community researchers; and I would like to see community researchers, in turn, take more seriously the tasks of deciding to whom they want to be useful and of measuring the usefulness of their research.

Of the four criteria in my first chapter, I am least worried about theories of knowledge in community research—not because they excel, but because they seem to be on a par with the social sciences as a whole, reflecting all the ambiguities and confusions of the day. I do think it is time to call a halt to criticizing logical positivism and to get on with more progressive contributions.

Even logical positivists acknowledged that the theory had died by the 1940s. Nothing has won widespread acceptance since. If anything, epistemological and methodological pluralism is the mark of the times, and the major challenge may be to be cognizant of this pluralism without letting it degenerate into an "anything goes" mode of operation. Nothing prevents such degeneration as much as mutual criticism, which is another good reason why the maturing of community research rests partly on changing any remaining norms that minimize such criticism in the field. As this chapter probably demonstrates, we will need practice to criticize in a way that is forceful but also sufficiently humble about recognizing one's own vulnerabilities. Criticism is psychologically and socially difficult—even in science, where it is purportedly welcomed and valued—and the tendency to be tolerant in the name of pluralism is deeply ingrained in our field. Hence, the social and psychological realities of science can butt heads with a critical epistemology in painful ways. However, the epistemological health of the field depends too much on this task not to make the effort and not to try to find forums and methods that make criticism a welcomed endeavor.

So far, I have leveled many criticisms at community research, particularly in contrast to program evaluation. As a result, the reader might ask whether the logical implication is that I think program evaluation has contributed more to social problem solving than to community psychology? At the risk of demonstrating my ignorance about the accomplishments of community research, I have to admit that I do hold that opinion. (Perhaps others can take up the challenge and show how wrong I am.) Those people with whom I have shared this speculation have reacted with understandable incredulity that I would even make this comparison, much less judge the outcome in favor of program evaluation. Such comparisons have to be made, however, if we are to take the task of judging the merits of community research seriously, for in comparing both the processes and the outcomes that characterize the two fields lies one of our best hopes for understanding how to improve them both.

I also have to admit that program evaluation has not done much to summarize or to disseminate its accomplishments, so incredulity is in some respects a reasonable response to my comment. First, therefore, let me mention some information about one of the best accomplishments that program evaluation has achieved, with the goal of encouraging us to take the contrast seriously. I will then go on to acknowledge some of the many difficulties that make such a comparison fraught with problems.

The U.S. General Accounting Office, an arm of Congress, has had a Program Evaluation and Methodology Division (PEMD) since 1980. With a staff of just over 100 evaluators, at any given time, PEMD is involved in about 45 ongoing studies. Some are self-initiated, but most are in response to Congressional requests about currently salient issues in social policy and programming, such as access to special education, CETA programs for disadvantaged adults, implications of block grants, costs and benefits of home health care, mandatory workfare programs, federal programs to improve pregnancy outcome, housing allowances, hazardous waste management, environmental quality, illegal aliens in the work force, and the impact of drinking-age laws on highway safety. PEMD evaluations routinely make a real difference in Congressional decisions that bear on a wide and plausible array of social-problem-solving criteria. For example, in 1984, Congress took away the Aid to Families With Dependent Children (AFDC) "earned income disregard." This "disregard" had previously allowed AFDC recipients to earn some money through jobs, with little or no reduction of AFDC benefits. Removing the disregard meant that recipients would lose AFDC benefits, including Medicaid, if they worked. The political left opposed removing the disregard for fear that such action would reduce overall income and force people back on welfare, but the political right supported it as a cost-saving measure that would have little bad effect and would encourage the work ethic. The PEMD evaluation showed that the political right was correct in important ways—people did not quit their jobs to return to welfare after the disregard was removed. Hence, Congress maintained the disregard removal. However, PEMD also showed that the political left had its valid points, too (notice value pluralism at work here)—removing the disregard led to important privations (especially in the South) for children, who lost Medicaid coverage. Hence, Congress extended Medicaid to people for one year after they left AFDC.

A huge national impact thus resulted from just one of a hundred studies by PEMD. PEMD's accomplishments stem in significant part from its careful attention to the four criteria for good social-problem-solving research that I outlined in my first chapter. PEMD bases its research strategies on sound understandings of how change occurs, of how research is used in policymaking, of the role of value pluralism in adjudicating policy debates, and of the kinds of knowledge that science can hope to contribute to that process. I am not sure that any contribution of community research to social problem solving would fare well in comparison to PEMD, and this is partly due, I assert, to its relative lack of attention to all of these four issues.

Having, I hope, intrigued you with this contrast, let me now acknowledge some of the difficulties in getting a clear answer to the question of the comparative merits of the two fields. First, I have stated the terms of the debate in a way that is consistent with my vision of the field—to address social problems in the sense discussed in my Chapter 2. Setting such terms is a fair challenge. But if the criterion were that of fostering a sense of "community identity," or of contributing to basic psychological theory, community research might fare best.

Second, a good answer to this question would have to use a multifaceted set of criteria that bear on social problem solving. These might include (a) the number and importance of the social problems studied, (b) improvements in existing practices and programs, (c) contributions to new policies that might significantly improve on old policies, (d) the number of dollars saved or earned, (e) conceptual influences on how the policy-shaping community thinks about the causes of and solutions to social problems, and (f) development of better theories about how to do research that contributes to social problem solving. The standard litany of caveats applies, of course: This list is incomplete, each criterion should be elaborated considerably to be useful, no criterion will be valid for all cases, and there is no single right way to measure each criterion, so that we should always try multiple ways of doing so. But, undoubtedly, the comparative merits of the two specialties would vary somewhat depending on exactly which criterion was used.

Third, the comparison is unfair in the important sense that hundreds of millions of dollars have been spent on program evaluation, and it directly or indirectly contributes to the work of a large number of professionals with direct access to all levels of social policy mechanisms in society. The nearest community psychology ever came to such a professional base was in community mental health centers, from which it has now largely withdrawn. The small academic base of community psychology cannot generate access and resources comparable to those of program evaluation. Given this discrepancy, in fact, if I were responding to my own argument I might try to make the case that community psychology was more cost-effective than program evaluation.

Fourth, it is not clear exactly what should count as community research and what should count as program evaluation. In the realm of prevention, for example, does community research get to count the major smoking prevention studies conducted mostly by psychologists specializing in behavioral medicine? Should we count Carol Weiss as a program evaluator because she is one of the major theorists in the field, or should we acknowledge that her primary identity might be as a sociologist and, so, not count her?

Finally, I deliberately chose to play to program evaluation's strengths by choosing to use PEMD as my example, for two reasons. One reason is the important rhetorical function of encouraging the reader to take the contrast seriously—if I picked the worst that program evaluation had to offer, would you still take the challenge seriously? The other reason is that, by comparing the best that a field has to offer, one gets a sense of its upper limits. It may take massive investment in a field to find out what those upper limits are; perhaps we would have a better sense of the upper limits of community research if it had received funding commensurate with program evaluation. Furthermore, if I examined the worst that each field has to offer, program evaluation might lose the comparison, for I have seen a good deal of incredibly bad work in that field. Finally, if I asked about the modal accomplishments of the two fields, program evaluation might win in absolute terms, given its massive resources and policy base—but, here, the cost-effectiveness issue becomes a real challenge.

In closing, I want to return briefly to an observation that I made earlier about the relative social structures of the two disciplines. I still think this is the key to many of the differences that I have discussed between the two fields. Perhaps, on reflection, community researchers will decide that the role they want to play is that of the academic gadfly who shows us possibilities for a better world that might be. Without a doubt, we need such researchers. We should make the decision to take that role consciously, however, and with due acknowledgment of the alternatives lost for social problem solving.

Even if my diagnosis is wrong, I hope that I have managed to raise some useful questions and to open a dialogue among different groups of researchers who really do share a good deal in common. We need to be talking with each other more about such matters, so that we can all learn how to do a better job of addressing the many pressing social problems that we all acknowledge need more attention.

CHAPTER 17

AN ASPIRATION FOR COMMUNITY RESEARCH

FERN CHERTOK, CHRISTOPHER KEYS,
PATRICK TOLAN, AND LEONARD JASON

The preceding chapters have addressed the full spectrum of issues and dilemmas that face the psychologist who chooses to do community research. However, although each section of this book has examined a particular aspect of the research process in depth, the result is neither a workbook nor a compendium of guidelines, and, in this regard, the reader who seeks specific instructions may be frustrated. Instead, and we believe, more significantly, what emerges from this conversation among researchers is a composite aspiration for the field of community research. An *aspiration* (as defined in Webster's New Collegiate Dictionary, 1976) is a "strong desire to achieve something high or great." Whereas guidelines describe the boundaries of a path and the immediate territory ahead, an aspiration represents the path's ultimate destination and, thus, imbues the journey with passion and dedication. The emergent aspiration to be described in this chapter is, in part, a reaffirmation of the fundamental spirit of Community Psychology as originally proposed at the 1965 Swampscott conference (Bennett et al., 1966; Price, Reinharz, Riger, & Wandersman, 1984) and again in Austin in 1975. Its key elements include an emphasis on exploring ecological factors that contribute to adaptive human functioning, a focus on action-oriented research that promotes community strengths, and a commitment to active collaboration with community members in all phases of the research process. What is new is the effort to give this aspiration substance by tying it to tangible implications for the content, structure, and process of community research. Without this important connection, an aspiration is no more than rhetoric.

Concepts such as *aspiration* or *mission* are seldom part of the official literature of Community Psychology (Cherniss & Krantz, 1983), although they frequently echo through private discussions and certainly form the backdrop for many conference presentations. Community psychology is still young in translating mission into action; however, it is not without models from which to learn. By studying one of the core aspirations of the Shaker movement we may better understand the integral role of community research's own coalescing mission:

> Do all your work as if you had a thousand years to live and as if you knew you must die tomorrow.   (Mother Ann Lee, Shaker founder)

Mother Ann Lee's injunction led her followers to form one of the most successful and influential communal societies in American history, and it has implications today for community research. Its paradoxical emphasis on the urgency of accomplishing important tasks and on taking the time needed to do a quality job is a reminder that although an aspiration gives meaning it does not simplify. As Davidson has pointed out in Chapter 12D, the purpose of a mission is not to camouflage the thorny issues but to draw them into the foreground and make clear why it is necessary to grapple with them. To work as if under an impending sentence of death is a constant reminder to focus our resources on the work that is deemed most important. The frustration of community researchers with the progress of the field over the past 20 years may, in part, be related to how often we have postponed asking the most central questions until some undefined time in the future when we will "know more" or be "more ready." Instead, Community Psychology in general and individual community researchers need to have the courage to set priorities for the field and then to act on them.

Setting an agenda for community research begins with the critical step of defining the phenomenon of interest. Although acknowledging the value of logical positivism, Kingry-Westergaard and Kelly (in Chapter 3) and Bry et al. (in Chapter 10) indicate the value of more active, flexible epistemologies such as constructivism and contextualism for identifying research assumptions more congruent with the quicksilver properties of community phenomena. More specifically, Seidman (in Chapter 9) has proposed that community research should turn its attention away from the study of individual and population attributes to a focus on describing, understanding, and changing social regularities. The term *social regularities* refers to the pattern and distribution of interactions or exchanges between individuals and the settings that they inhabit or between settings or mesosystems themselves. In a similar vein, Lorion (in Chapter 4) used the term *transaction* to capture the reciprocal, ongoing, and evolving exchange between the individual and the environment. This concept adds a temporal dimension to our understanding of the development of individual and of aggregate behavior in a setting and may highlight critical points at which prevention efforts will be most effective. Although particular constructs may need further refinement, these and other authors in this volume (e.g., Hobfoll) are pushing the field to develop a vocabulary for thinking about community phenomena that is not person-centered. As Allen pointed out in Chapter 12B, language plays a pivotal role in defining what we see and the questions that we can ask. Committing the field to an extraindividual, relational language will help to ensure a continuing focus on people embedded in settings.

The Shaker aspiration makes it clear that choosing what needs to be done is only the first step. Integrity of purpose requires dedication to doing the best job possible. To do one's work as if time were not a factor liberates the craftsperson and the researcher alike to proceed with thoughtful planning and scrutinizing attention to detail. Freedom from the pressure of a market economy and from conventional taste allowed the Shakers to create their distinctive slat-back chair. Its deceptive simplicity is the result of long trial and error in determining, among other things, the pattern of spacing between slats that makes the back appear suspended in air above the seat and legs.

Many of the authors in this book have voiced a similar plea for the careful construction and testing of theory in community research. Shinn (in Chapter 11) has cogently and compellingly called attention to the necessity of developing nomological networks that include a designation of the relevant level or levels of analysis for each proposed construct. She further prompts us to follow through by selecting or designing measures that neither bypass the relevant level of analysis for an easier source of data (i.e., the individual) nor mix levels as if they were qualitatively interchangeable. Several chapters have described available and potential measurement strategies. Drawing on strategies of research in the humanities, Levine (in Chapter 13C) describes the use of historical and investigative reporting in weaving together multiple perspectives. Both Cherniss (in Chapter 12C) and Maton (in Chapter 13B) discuss the role of qualitative methodology in the generation and testing of hypotheses and clearly state that these strategies should not be thought of as an easy way around the difficult work of research. Viable standards for rigor in use of qualitative methods can be adapted from those used in other fields, such as sociology. From a different perspective, Rapkin and Mulvey (in Chapter 13A) question the present attitude of community research toward quantitative methods. Just as the selection of qualitative methods needs to be carefully thought out, these authors suggest that it is necessary to evaluate how well our research questions adhere to the assumptions and limits of various quantitative methods. The result of this deliberation may be the development of quantitative strategies that fit the unique demands of our phenomena of interest.

Finally, the Shaker aspiration reminds us that just as our values shape the work to which we set our minds and hands, so, in turn, the work will shape us. Shaker craftspeople made everyday objects that have a striking yet staid beauty. Shaker handwork is distinctive in its elegant simplicity and practicality. Less tangible, but no less significant, is the impact of the work on the artisans themselves. The challenge of designing a basket or chair that embodies a belief in humility, orderliness, and the equality of the sexes forces the craftsperson to explore the complex meaning and application of those values. Shakers were involved in an ongoing encounter with the implications of their values that brought life to those beliefs.

Community Psychology will also profit from struggling to implement its cohering aspiration. Collaboration, participation, and empowerment are repeated themes in this volume. Serrano-García (in Chapter 14) and Swift (in Chapter 15E) have defined a set of necessary and sufficient conditions for collaboration and participation. According to these authors, and to Robinson (Chapter 15D) and Riger (Chapter 5), the underlying challenge of developing truly horizontal relationships with research participants lies in our willingness to accept the validity of the constructed reality of community members. By giving voice to groups and individuals in devalued roles, such as mental patients or line workers, we are enacting respect for their diverse talents and perspective. In a similar vein, Rappaport (Chapter 6) and Fawcett (Chapter 7) make it clear that empowerment is not only a phenomenon of interest, but also a foundational belief about one's relationship with others. It is a stance that demands that research endeavor, in its separate parts and in total, to address issues that are defined by the community, to afford the possibility of successful and sustainable change, and to enhance the control that traditionally marginal groups have over their lives.

The level of participation and respect that these authors are requiring of community research will not be easy to implement. Bond (Chapter 15A) has elaborated on the seemingly unavoidable differences in power and resources that exist between community researchers and community members. Community psychology is firmly rooted in the institution of academics, which often reinforces the use of a few narrow dimensions for evaluating worth—unfortunately, dimensions on which most unempowered groups fall short. To engage honestly in horizontal relations with community members, community psychologists will have to free themselves from this powerful bias and explore many dimensions on which they may not fare as well. The very struggle to live up to the values of empowerment and collaboration cannot help but teach us about the varied and complex meaning of those values. Having placed themselves in a position of equal partnership, community psychologists will better understand the challenging task facing community settings and organizations that attempt to collaborate or contemplate changing their internal distribution of power and decision making.

To live according to their beliefs, the Shakers found it necessary to form separate communities where the pattern and structure of daily life were under their control. I hope that community psychology will not have to take so drastic a step in order to fulfill its own aspiration. Cauce (Chapter 16B) reminds us that logical positivism and the traditional research paradigm of psychology are not without merit in evaluating community programs. However, at the same time, community psychology cannot expect to continue without making some changes in its own social regularities. Repucci (Chapter 13D) proposes deritualizing those habits of community research that have become sacred through repetition. He suggests that we need to change or expand the consensually accepted method in ways that correspond to the central questions of the field. Toward this end, Feis (Chapter 16A) has made a series of specific suggestions about how graduate students should be educated and indoctrinated into the content and culture of community research. She proposes that the structure of graduate education be changed to include input from diverse sources, including community members and faculty from other disciplines, collaborative projects that involve faculty and students working together in all phases of the research process, and hiring of new faculty on the basis of more than the number of publications on their vita. Finally, Cauce has requested that senior faculty, rather than junior faculty or graduate students, lead the way by transforming their own programs of research so that they more closely approach the aspirations of the field.

Long after its heyday, the fidelity with which Shaker life reflected Shaker belief still makes an impression. The enduring legacy of Shaker life is still evident in American culture and thought, and Shaker pragmatism has become part of the American idiom. As the field of community research converses, grapples with, and struggles toward its own aspiration, we hope that it will continue to exceed its boundaries and have a constructive impact on the larger discipline of psychology and on social problem solving.

REFERENCES

Adler, M. J. (1987), *We hold these truths: Understanding the ideas and ideals of the Constitution*. New York: Macmillan.

Agar, M. H. (1980). *The professional stranger: An informal introduction to ethnography.* New York: Academic Press.

Alinsky, S. D. (1969). *Reveille for radicals*. New York: Vintage Books.

Allport, F. H. (1962). A structuronomic conception of behavior: Individual and collective. I. Structural theory and the master problem of social psychology. *Journal of Abnormal and Personality Psychology, 64,* 3–30.

Altman, I. (1987). Community psychology twenty years later: Still another crisis in psychology. *American Journal of Community Psychology, 15,* 613–627.

Altman, I., & Rogoff, B. (1987). World views in psychology: Trait, interactional, organismic and transactional perspectives. In D. Stokols & I. Altman (Eds.), *Handbook of environmental psychology* (pp. 7–40). New York: Wiley.

Alvarez, S. (1980). *Definición de liderato de una comunidad puertorequeña*. Unpublished master's thesis. University of Puerto Rico, Rio Piedras.

American Psychological Association. (1982). *Ethical principles in the conduct of research with human participants*. Washington, DC: Author.

Antonovsky, A. (1979). *Health, stress, and coping*. New York: Jossey-Bass.

Aronson, E. (1978). *The jigsaw classroom*. Beverly Hills, CA: Sage.

Ash, M. G., & Woodward, W. R. (Eds.) (1988). *Psychology in twentieth-century thought and society.* New York: Cambridge University Press.

Baer, D. M., Wolf, M. M., & Risley, T. R. (1968). Some current dimensions of applied behavior analysis. *Journal of Applied Behavior Analysis. 1,* 91–97.

Baer, D. M., Wolf, M. M., & Risley, T. R. (1987). Some still-current dimensions of applied behavior analysis. *Journal of Applied Behavior Analysis, 20,* 313–327.

Barker, R. G. (1960). Ecology and motivation. In M. R. Jones (Ed.), *Nebraska Symposium on Motivation* (pp. 1–49). Lincoln: University of Nebraska Press.

Barker, R. G. (1968). *Ecological psychology: Concepts and methods for studying the environment of human behavior.* Stanford, CA: Stanford University Press.

Barker, R. G. (1987a). Explorations in ecological psychology. In R. G. Barker, *Midwest Psychological Field Station*. Lawrence: University of Kansas.

Barker, R. G. (1987b). Prospecting in environmental psychology: Oskaloosa revisited. In D. Stokols & I. Altman (Eds.), *Handbook of environmental psychology* (pp. 1413–1432). New York: Wiley.

Barker, R. G., & Gump, P. V. (1964). *Big school, small school: High school size and student behavior.* Stanford, CA: Stanford University Press.

Barlow, D., Hayes, S., & Nelson, R. (1984). *The scientist practitioner: Research and accountability in clinical and educational settings*. New York: Pergamon.

Bateson, G. (1972). *Steps to an ecology of the mind.* San Francisco: Chandler.

Bateson, G. (1979). *Mind and nature: A necessary unity.* New York: Bantam.

Beauchamp, T. L. (1982). *Philosophical ethics: An introduction to moral philosophy.* New York: McGraw-Hill.

Becker, H. (1967). Whose side are we on? *Social Problems, 14* (Winter), 239–247.

Belenky, M. F., Clinchy, B. M., Goldberger, N. R., & Tarule, J. M. (1986). *Women's ways of knowing: The development of self, voice and mind.* New York: Basic Books.

Bennett, C. C., Anderson, L. S., Cooper, S., Hassol, L., Klein, D. C., & Rosenblum, G. (Eds.). (1966). *Community psychology: A report of the Boston conference of the education of psychologists for community mental health.* Boston: Boston University Press.

Berg, D. N., & Smith, K. K. (Eds.). (1988). *The self in social inquiry: Research methods.* Beverly Hills: Sage.

Berger, P., & Luckmann, T. (1967). *The social construction of reality.* New York: Doubleday.

Bergin, A. E., (1966). Some implications of psychotherapy research for therapeutic practice. *Journal of Abnormal Psychology, 71,* 235–246.

Berk, R. A., & Rossi, P. H. (1977). Doing good or worse: Evaluation research politically reexamined. In G. V. Glass (Ed.), *Evaluation Studies Review Annual, 2,* 77–89.

Berman, P., & McLaughlin, M. W. (1978). *Federal programs supporting educational change: Vol. 8. Implementing and sustaining innovations* (Contract No. R-1589/8-HEW). Washington, DC: U.S. Office of Education.

Bernal, G., Serrano-García, I., Alvarez, A., & Ribera, J. (1989). *Participatory needs assessment of employees at the University of Puerto Rico.* Unpublished manuscript.

Billings, A., & Moos, R. (1982). Work stress and the stress-buffering role of work and family resources. *Journal of Occupational Behavior, 3,* 215–232.

Blakely, C. H., Mayer, J. P., Gottschalk, R. G., Schmitt, N., Davidson, W. S., Roitman, D. B., & Emshoff, J. G. (1987). The fidelity–adaptation debate: Implications for the implementation of public sector social programs. *American Journal of Community Psychology, 15,* 253–268.

Bleir, R. (1984). *Science and gender: A critique of biology and its theories on women.* Elmsford, NY: Pergamon Press.

Blumer, H. (1969). *Symbolic interactionism: Perspective and method.* Englewood Cliffs, NJ: Prentice-Hall.

Bogat, G. A., & Jason, L. A. (in press). Dogs bark at those they do not recognize: Toward an integration of behaviorism and community psychology. In J. Rappaport & E. Seidman (Eds.), *Handbook of community psychology.* New York: Plenum.

Bolman, L. G., & Deal, T. E. (1984). *Modern approaches to understanding organizations.* San Francisco: Jossey-Bass.

Borkman, T. (1990). Experiential, professional and lay frames of reference. In T. J. Powell (Ed.), *Working with self-help.* Silver Spring, MD: National Association of Social Workers.

Bouchard, T. J., Jr. (1976). Field research methods. In M. D. Dunnette (Ed.), *Handbook of industrial and organizational psychology* (pp 363–413). Chicago: Rand-McNally.

Boyte, H. C., & Reissman, F. (Eds.). (1986). *The new populism: The politics of empowerment.* Philadelphia : Temple University Press.

Brim, O., Glass, D., Lavin, D., & Goodman, N. (1962). *Personality and decision processes: Studies in the social psychology of thinking.* Palo Alto, CA: Stanford University Press.

Bronfenbrenner, U. (1977). Toward an experimental ecology of human development. *American Psychologist, 32,* 513–531.

Bronfenbrenner, U. (1979). *The ecology of human development.* Cambridge, MA: Harvard University Press.

Bronfenbrenner, U. (1986). Ecology of the family as a context for human development: Research perspectives. *Developmental Psychology, 22,* 723–742.

Brown, G. W., & Harris, T. (1978). *Social origins of depression: A study of psychiatric disorder in women.* New York: Free Press.

Brown, L. D. (1983). Organizing participatory research: Interfaces for joint inquiry and organizational change. *Journal of Occupational Behavior, 4,* 9–19.

Brown, L. D., & Tandon, R. (1983). Ideology and political economy in inquiry: Action research and participatory research. *Journal of Applied Behavioral Science, 19*(3), 177–194.

Brown, R. D. (1968). Manipulation of the environmental press in a college residence hall. *Personnel and Guidance Journal, 46,* 555-560.

Bryk, A. S. (1983). *Stakeholder-based evaluation.* San Francisco: Jossey-Bass.

Calsyn, R. J., Tornatzky, L. G., & Dittmar, S. (1977). Incomplete adoption of an innovation: The case of goal attainment scaling. *Evaluation, 4,* 127–130.

Cameron, K. S. (1986). Effectiveness as paradox: Consensus and conflict in conceptions of organizational effectiveness. *Management Science, 32,* 539–553.

Campbell, D. T. (1988). *Methodology and epistemology for social science: Selected papers.* Chicago, University of Chicago Press.

Campbell, D. T., & Fiske, D. W. (1959). Convergent and discriminant validation by the multitrait–multimethod matrix. *Psychological Bulletin, 56,* 81–105.

Campbell, D. T., & Stanley, J. C. (1963). *Experimental and quasi-experimental designs for research.* Chicago: Rand-McNally.

Campbell, J. P. (1977). The cutting edge of leadership: An overview. In J. G. Hunt & L. L. Larson (Eds.), *Leadership: The cutting edge* (pp. 221–234). Carbondale: Southern Illinois University Press.

Castañeda, I., Domenech, N., & Figueroa, O. (1987). *Una identificación de necesidades y recursos en las personas deambulantes de Santurce.* Unpublished master's thesis. University of Puerto Rico, Rio Piedras.

Chalmers, A. F. (1976). *What is this thing called science?* St. Lucia, Australia: University of Queensland Press.

Chaplin, J. S., & Krawiec, T. S. (1979). *Systems and theories of psychology.* (4th ed.). New York: Holt, Rinehart & Winston.

Chavis, D., Stucky, P. E., & Wandersman, A. (1983). Returning research to the community: A relationship between scientist and citizen. *American Psychologist, 38,* 424–434.

Chavis, D., & Wandersman, A. (1986). Roles for researcher and the researched in neighborhood development. In R. Taylor (Ed.), *Urban neighborhoods: Research and policy* (pp. 215–249). New York: Praeger.

Chein, I. (1954). The environment as a determinant of behavior. *Journal of Social Psychology, 39,* 115–127.

Cherniss, C., & Krantz, D. (1983) The ideological community as an antidote to burnout in the human services. In B. Farber (Ed.), *Stress and burnout in the human service professions* (pp. 198–212). New York: Pergamon Press.

Cherniss, D. (1980). *Professional burnout in human services organizations.* New York: Praeger.

Chicago Foundation for Women (March 30, 1988). Women's Leadership Development & Initiative [Minutes of advisory committee].

Churchman, C. W. (1971). *The design of inquiring systems.* New York: Basic Books.

Clark, K. B., & Clark, M. P. (1939). The development of consciousness of self in the emergence of racial identification in Negro pre-school children. *Journal of Social Psychology, 10,* 591–597.

Clark, K. B., & Clark, M. P. (1947). Racial identification and preferences in Negro children. In T. M. Newcomb & E. L. Hartley (Eds.). *Readings in social psychology* (pp. 169–178) New York: Holt, Rinehart & Winston.

Coleman, J. S. (1972). *Policy research in the social sciences.* Morristown, NJ: General Learning Press.

Colon, A. (1982). *Los desempleados: Estudio etnográfico sobre la problemática personal y su visión del desempleo en Pueto Rico.* Unpublished master's thesis. University of Puerto Rico, Rio Piedras.

Cook, T. D. (1983). Quasi-experimentation: Its ontology, epistemology, and methodology. In G. Morgan (Ed.), *Beyond method: Strategies for social research* (pp. 74–94). Beverly Hills, CA: Sage.

Cook, T. D. (1986). Postpositivist critical multiplism. In L. Shotland & M. M. Mark (Eds.), *Social science and social policy* (pp. 21–62). Beverly Hills, CA. Sage.

Cook, T. D., & Campbell, D. T. (1979). *Quasi-experimentation: Design and analysis issues for field settings.* Chicago: Rand McNally.

Cook, T. D., Levinson-Rose, J., & Pollard, W. E. (1980). The misutilization of evaluation findings: Some conceptual pitfalls. *Knowledge: Creation, Dissemination, Utilization, 1,* 477–498.

Cook, T. D., & Shadish, W. R., Jr. (1986). Program evaluation: The worldly science. *Annual Review of Psychology, 37,* 193–232.

Cowen, E. L. (1973). Social and community interventions. *Annual Review of Psychology, 24,* 423–472.

Cowen, E. L. (1980). The wooing of primary prevention. *American Journal of Community Psychology, 8,* 258–284.

Cronbach, L. J. (1975). Beyond the two disciplines of scientific psychology. *American Psychologist, 30,* 116–127.

Cronbach, L. J. (1982a). *Designing evaluations of educational and social programs.* San Francisco: Jossey-Bass.

Cronbach, L. J. (1982b). Prudent aspirations for social inquiry. In W. K. Kruskal (Ed.), *The social sciences: Their nature and uses.* Chicago: University of Chicago Press.

Cronbach, L. J. (1986). Social inquiry by and for earthlings. In D. W. Fiske & R. A. Shweder (Eds.), *Metatheory in social science: Pluralisms and subjectives* (pp. 93–107). Chicago: University of Chicago Press.

Cronbach, L. J., & Meehl, P. E. (1955). Construct validity in psychological tests. *Psychological Bulletin, 52,* 281–302.

D'Andrade, R. (1986). Three scientific world views and the covering law model. In D. W. Fiske & R. A. Shweder (Eds.), *Metatheory in social science: Pluralisms and subjectives* (pp. 19–41). Chicago: University of Chicago Press.

D'Aunno, T., Klein, D., & Susskind, E. (1985). Seven approaches for the study of community phenomena. In E. Susskind & D. Klein (Eds.), *Community research: Methods, paradigms, and applications* (pp. 421–495). New York: Praeger.

D'Aunno, T., & Price, R. (1984a). The context and objectives of community research. In K. Heller, R. Price, S. Reinhartz, S. Riger, & A. Wandersman (Eds.), *Psychology and community change: Challenges of the future* (pp. 51–67). Homewood, IL: Dorsey Press.

D'Aunno, T., & Price, R. (1984b). Methodologies in community research: Analytic and action approaches. In K. Heller, R. Price, S. Reinhartz, S. Riger, & A. Wandersman (Eds.), *Psychology and community change: Challenges of the future.* Homewood, IL: Dorsey Press.

Dalton, J. H., Elias, M. J., & Howe, G. W. (1985). Studying the emerging community of community psychology. In E. C. Susskind & D. C. Klein (Eds.), *Community research: Methods, paradigms, and applications* (pp. 106–138). New York: Praeger.

Dansereau, F., Jr., Alutto, J. A., Markham, S. E., & Dumas, M. (1982). Multiplexed supervision and leadership: An application of within and between analysis. In J. G. Hunt, U. Sekaran, & C. A. Schriesheim (Eds.), *Leadership: Beyond establishment views* (pp. 81–103). Carbondale: Southern Illinois University Press.

Dansereau, F., Alutto, J. A., & Yammarino, F. J. (1984). *Theory testing in organizational behavior: The variant approach.* Englewood Cliffs, NJ: Prentice-Hall.

Dansereau, F., & Markham, S. E. (1987). Levels of analysis in personnel and human resources management. *Personnel and Human Resources Management, 5,* 1–50.

Davidson, W. S., Redner, R., & Saul, J. (1983). Models of measuring social and community change. In E. Seidman (Ed.), *Handbook of social intervention* (pp. 99–118). Beverly Hills, CA: Sage.

Dobson, D., & Cook, T. J. (1980). Avoiding Type III error in program evaluation: Results from a field experiment. *Evaluation and Program Planning, 3,* 269–276.

Dohrenwend, B. S., Krasnoff, L., Askenasy, A. R., & Dohrenwend, B. P. (1978). Exemplification of a method for scaling life events: The PERI Life Events Scale. *Journal of Health and Social Behavior, 19,* 205–229.

Dollard, J. (1957). *Caste and class in a southern town.* Garden City, NJ: Doubleday/Anchor.

Edelstein, M. R. (1988). *Contaminated communities: The social and psychological impacts of residential toxic exposure.* Boulder, CO: Westview Press.

Efran J. S., Lukens, R. J., & Lukens, M. D. (1988). Constructivism: What's in it for you? *The Family Therapy Networker* (September/October).

Eisenberg, G., & DeMaso, D. R. (1985). Fifty Years of the American Journal of Orthopsychiatry: An overview and introduction. In E. Flaxman (Ed.), *American Journal of Orthopsychiatry: Annotated index. Vols. 1–50. 1930–1980.* Greenwich, CT: JAI Press.

Elias, M. J., Dalton, J. H., Franco, R., & Howe, G. W. (1984). Academic and nonacademic community psychologists: An analysis of divergence is settings, roles, and values. *American Journal of Community Psychology, 12,* 281–302.

Elias, M., Gara, M., & Ubriaco, M. (1985). Sources of stress and support in children's transition to middle school: An empirical analysis. *Journal of Clinical Child Psychology, 14,* 112–118.

Elliot, G. (1975). *Cómo ayudar a los grupos a tomar decisiónes.* Mexico City: Ediciones Diana.

Emshoff, J. G., Blakely, C., Gottschalk, R., Mayer, J., Davidson, W. S., & Erickson, S. (1987). Innovation in education and criminal justice: Measuring fidelity of implementation and program effectiveness. *Educational Evaluation and Policy Analysis, 9,* 300–311.

Fairweather, G. W. (1967). *Methods for experimental social innovation.* New York, Wiley.

Fairweather, G. W. (1980). Community psychology for the 1980s and beyond. *Evaluation and Program Planning, 3,* 245–250.

Fairweather, G. W., & Davidson, W. (1986) *Community experimentation: Theory, methods, and practice.* New York: McGraw Hill.

Fairweather, G. W., Sanders, D. H., Cressler, D. F., Maynard, H., & Bleck, D. S. (1969). *Community life for the mentally ill.* Chicago: Aldine.

Falicov, C. J. (1988). Learning to think culturally, In H. A. Liddle, D. Breunlin, R. Schwartz (Eds.), *The handbook of family therapy training and supervision* (pp. 335–337). New York: Guilford Press.

Fals-Borda, O., & Rodriguez, C. (1985). *Investigación participativa.* Montevideo, Uruguay: Ediciónes de la Banda Oriental.

Fawcett, S. B., Mathews, R. M., & Fletcher, R. K. (1980). Some promising dimensions for behavioral community technology. *Journal of Applied Behavior Analysis, 13,* 508–518.

Fawcett, S. B., Seekins, T., & Jason, L. A. (1987). Policy research and child passenger safety legislation: A case study and experimental evaluation. *Journal of Social Issues, 43,* 133–148.

Fawcett, S. B., Seekins, T., & Silber, L. (1988). Low-income voter registration: A small-scale evaluation of an agency-based voter registration strategy. *American Journal of Community Psychology, 16,* 751–758.

Fawcett, S. B., Seekins, T., Whang, P. L., Muiu, C., & Suarez de Balcazar, Y. (1982). Involving consumers in decision making. *Social Policy, 13,* 36–41.

Fawcett, S. B., Seekins, T., Whang, P. L., Muiu, C., & Suarez de Balcazar, Y. (1984). Creating and using social technologies for community empowerment. In J. Rappaport, C. Swift, & R. Hess (Eds.), *Studies in empowerment: Steps toward understanding and action* (pp. 145–172). New York: Haworth Press.

Fawcett, S. B., Suarez de Balcazar, Y., Whang-Ramos, P. L., Seekins, T., Bradford, B., & Mathews, R. M. (1988). The Concerns Report: Involving consumers in planning for rehabilitation and independent living services. *American Rehabilitation, 14,* 17–19.

Felner, R. D., & Adan, A. M. (1988). The School Transitional Environment Project: An ecological intervention and evaluation. In R. H. Price, E. L. Cowen, R. P. Lorion, & J. Ramos-McKay (Eds.), *14 ounces of prevention: A casebook for practitioners.* (pp. 111–122). Washington, DC: American Psychological Association.

Felner, R. D., Ginter, G., & Primavera, J. (1982). Primary prevention during school transitions: Social support and environmental structure. *American Journal of Community Psychology, 10,* 277–290.

Feyerabend, P. (1975). *Against method.* London: New Left Books.

Feyerabend, P. (1978). *Science in a free society* (pp. 73–107). London: New Left Books.

Firebaugh, G. (1980). Groups as contexts and frog ponds. In K. H. Roberts & L. Burstein (Eds.), *Issues in aggregation: New directions for methodology of social and behavioral science* (Vol. 6, pp. 43–52). San Francisco: Jossey-Bass.

Fish, V. K. (1983). Feminist scholarship in sociology: An emerging research model. *Wisconsin Sociologist, 20,* 45–56.

Fishman, D., & Neigher, W. (1982). American psychology in the eighties: Who will buy? *American Psychologist, 37,* 533–546.

Fiske, D. W., & Shweder, R. A. (Eds.). (1986). *Metatheory in social science: Pluralisms and subjectivities.* Chicago: University of Chicago Press.

Flax, J. (1983). Political philosophy and the patriarchal unconscious: A psychoanalytic perspective on epistemology and metaphysics. In S. Harding & M. B. Hintikka (Eds.), *Discovering reality: Feminist perspectives on epistemology, metaphysics, methodology, and the philosophy of science* (pp. 245–281). London: Reidel.

Florin, P., Giamartino, G. A., Kenny, D. A., & Wandersman, A. (1988). *Uncovering climate and group influence by separating individual and group effects.* Unpublished manuscript, University of Rhode Island.

Frederickson, N. (1972). Toward a taxonomy of situations. *American Psychologist, 27,* 114–123.

Freedman, J. (1973). The tyranny of structurelessness. In A. Koedt, E. Levine, & A. Rapino (Eds.), *Radical feminism* (pp. 285–299). New York: Quadrangle.

French, J., & Raven, B. (1972). The bases of social power. In D. Cartwright & A. Zander (Eds.), *Group dynamics: Research and theory* (2nd ed., pp. 607–623). New York: Row & Peterson.

French, J. R. P., Jr., Rodgers, W., & Cobb, S. (1974). Adjustment as person–environment fit. In G. V. Coelho, D. A. Hamburg, & J. E. Adams (Eds.), *Coping and adaptation* (pp. 316–333). New York: Basic Books.

Fuller, S. (1988). *Social epistemology.* Bloomington: Indiana University Press.

Gaernter, S. L., & Dovidio, J. F. (Eds.). (1987). *Prejudice, discrimination, and racism.* Orlando, FL: Academic Press.

Garbarino, J., & Sherman, D. (1980). High-risk neighborhoods and high-risk families: The human ecology of child maltreatment. *Child Development, 51,* 188–198.

Gatz, M., & Liem, R. (1977). Social change: II. Systems analysis and intervention. In I. Iscoe, B. Bloom, & C. D. Spielberger (Eds.), *Community psychology in transition* (pp. 117–122). Washington, DC: Hemisphere.

Geertz, C. (1973). *The interpretation of cultures.* New York: Basic Books.

Geller, E. S. (1984). A delayed reward strategy for large-scale motivation of safety belt use: A test of long-term impact. *Accident Analysis and Prevention, 16,* 457–463.

Gergen, K. J. (1982). *Toward transformation in social knowledge.* New York: Springer-Verlag.

Gergen, K. (1985). The social constructionist movement in social psychology. *American Psychologist 40*(3), 266–275.

Gesten, E., & Jason, L. (1987). Social and community interventions. *American Review of Psychology, 38,* 427–460.

Gibran, K. (1923). *The prophet.* New York: Knopf.

Giere, R. N. (1988). *Explaining science: A cognitive approach.* Chicago: The University of Chicago Press.

Gilligan, C. (1982). *In a different voice.* Cambridge, MA: Harvard University Press.

Gilmore, D. C., Beehr, T. A., & Richter, D. J. (1979). Effects of leader behaviors on subordinate performance and satisfaction: A laboratory experiment with student employees. *Journal of Applied Psychology, 64,* 166–172.

Glaser, B., & Strauss, A. L. (1967). *The discovery of grounded theory: Strategies for qualitative research.* Chicago: Aldine.

Gleick, J. (1987). *Chaos: Making a new science.* New York: Penguin.

Glick, W. (1980). Problems in cross-level inferences. In K. H. Roberts & L. Burstein (Eds.), *Issues in aggregation: New directions for methodology of social and behavioral science* (Vol. 6, pp. 17–30). San Francisco: Jossey-Bass.

Glick, W. H. (1985). Conceptualizing and measuring organizational and psychological climate: Pitfalls in multilevel research. *Academy of Management Review, 10,* 601–616.

Glick, W. H. (1988). Response: Organizations are not central tendencies: Shadowboxing in the dark, Round 2. *Academy of Management Review, 13,* 133–137.

Glick, W. H., & Roberts, K. H. (1984). Hypothesized interdependence, assumed independence. *Academy of Management Review, 9,* 722–735.

Glidewell, J. C. (1966). Perspectives in community mental health. In C. C. Bennett, L. S. Anderson, L. Hassol, D. C. Klein, & G. Rosenblum (Eds.), *Community psychology: A report of the Boston conference on the education of psychologists for community mental health* (pp. 33–49). Boston: Boston University Press.

Goffman, E. (1961). *Asylums.* Garden City, NJ: Doubleday.

Goldberger, N. R., Clinchy, B. M., Belenky, M. F., & Tarule, J. M. (1986). *Women's ways of knowing: On gaining a voice.* In P. Shaver & C. Hendrick (Eds.), *Sex and gender* (pp. 201–225). Beverly Hills, CA: Sage.

Goldenberg, I. I. (1970). *Build me a mountain: Youth, poverty, and the creation of new settings.* Cambridge, MA: MIT Press.

Golembiewski, R. T., Billingsley, K., & Yeager, J. (1976). Measuring change and persistence in human affairs: Types of change generated by OD designs. *Journal of Applied Behavioral Science, 12,* 133–157.

Goodstein, L. D., & Sandler, I. (1978). Using psychology to promote human welfare: A conceptual analysis of the role of community psychology. *American Psychologist, 33,* 882–892.

Gottman, J. (1979). *Marital interaction.* New York: Academic Press.

Gould, S. J. (1981). *The mismeasure of man.* New York: Norton.

Graen, G. B., Novak, M. A., & Sommerkamp, P. (1982). The effects of leader–member exchange and job design on productivity and satisfaction: Testing a dual attachment model. *Organizational Behavior and Human Performance, 30,* 109–131.

Group for the Advancement of Psychiatry. (1959). *Some observations on controls in psychiatric research* (Report No. 42). New York: Author.

Gruber, J., & Trickett, E. J. (1987). Can we empower others? The paradox of empowerment in the governing of an alternative public school. *American Journal of Community Psychology, 15,* 353–371.

Guion, R. M. (1973). A note on organizational climate. *Organizational Behavior and Human Performance, 9,* 120–125.

Hall, A. R. (1966). *The scientific revolution 1500–1800: The formation of the modern scientific attitude* (2nd ed., pp. 159–185). Boston: Beacon Press.

Hall, G. E., & Hord, S. M. (1987). *Change in schools: Facilitating the process.* Albany, NY: State University of New York Press.

Hall, R. J. (1988). *A level of analysis approach to construct validity and relationship issues in perceived climate and job satisfaction measures.* Unpublished doctoral dissertation, University of Maryland.

Harding, S. (1986). *The science question in feminism.* Ithaca, NY: Cornell University Press.

Harding, S. (Ed.), (1987). Introduction: Is there a feminist method? In S. Harding (Ed.), *Feminism and methodology.* Bloomington: University of Indiana Press.

Harding, S., & Hintikka, M. B. (1983). *Discovering reality: Feminist perspectives on epistemology, metaphysics, methodology, and the philosophy of science.* London: Reidel.

Harding, S., & O'Barr, J. F. (1987). *Sex and scientific inquiry.* Chicago: University of Chicago Press.

Hare-Mustin, R. T., & Marecek, J. (1988). The meaning of difference: Gender, theory, postmodernism and psychology. *American Psychologist, 43,* 455–464.

Harre, R. (1981). The positivist–empiricist approach and its alternative. In P. Reason & J. Rowan (Eds.), *Human inquiry: A sourcebook of new paradigm research* (pp. 3–35). New York: Wiley.

Hartsock, N. C. M. (1983). The feminist standpoint: Developing the ground for a specifically feminist historical materialism. In S. Harding & M. B. Hintikka (Eds.), *Discovering reality: Feminist perspectives on epistemology, metaphysics, methodology, and the philosophy of science* (pp. 283–310). London: Reidel.

Hazel, K. L. (1988). Community psychology and creativity: A call for oneness. *Community Psychologist, 21*(3), 24.

Heidbreder, E. (1933). *Seven psychologies.* New York: Appleton.

Heller, K. (1988). *The return to community.* Invited Address presented to the division of Community Psychology at the 96th annual meeting of the American Psychological Association, Atlanta, GA, August 1988.

Heller, K., & Monahan, J. (1977). *Psychology and social change.* Homewood, IL: Dorsey Press.

Heller, K., Price, R., Reinharz, S., Riger, S., & Wandersman, A. (1984). *Psychology and community change: Challenges of the future* (2nd ed.). Homewood, IL: Dorsey Press.

Hesse, M. B. (1966). *Models and analogies in science.* Notre Dame, IN: University of Notre Dame Press.

Hinrichsen, G. A., Revenson, T. A., & Shinn, M. (1985). Does self-help help? An empirical investigation of scoliosis peer support groups. *Journal of Social Issues, 41,* 65–87.

Hirsch, B., & Rapkin, B. D. (1986). Social networks and adult social identities. *American Journal of Community Psychology 14*(4), 395–412.

Hoffman, L. (1981). *Foundations of family therapy: A conceptual framework for systems change.* New York: Basic Books.

Howard, G. (1985). The role of values in the science of psychology. *American Psychologist, 40,* 255–265.

Humphreys, P. (Ed.). (1986). Causality in the social sciences [Special Issue]. *Synthese, 68.*

Hunter, A., & Ringer, S. (1986). The meaning of community in community mental health. *Journal of Community Psychology, 14,* 55–71.

Ilgen, D. R., & Fujii, D. S. (1976). An investigation of the validity of leader behavior descriptions obtained from subordinates. *Journal of Applied Psychology, 61,* 642–651.

Irizarry, A. (1978). *Hacia una identificación de necesidades en la comunidad de Buen Consejo.* Unpublished master's thesis. University of Puerto Rico, Rio Piedras.

Irizarry, A., & Serrano-García, I. (1979). Intervención en la investigación: Su aplicación en el Barrio Buen Consejo, Rio Piedras, Puerto Rico, *Boletín de AVEPSO, 2,* 6–21.

James, L. R. (1982). Aggregation bias in estimates of perceptual agreement. *Journal of Applied Psychology, 67,* 219–229.

James, L. R., Joyce, W. F., & Slocum, J. W., Jr. (1988). Comment: Organizations do not cognize. *Academy of Management Review, 13,* 129–132.

James, L. R., & Sells, S. B. (1981). Psychological climate: Theoretical perspectives and empirical research. In D. Magnusson (Ed.), *Toward a psychology of situations: An interactional approach* (pp. 275–295). Hillsdale, NJ: Erlbaum.

Jason, L. A. (1989). *Eco-transactional behavioral research.* DePaul University. Manuscript submitted for publication.

Jason, L. A., Betts, D., Johnson, J., Smith, S., Kruckeberg, S., & Cradock, M. (1989). An evaluation of an orientation plus tutoring school-based prevention program. *Professional School Psychology, 4,* 273–284.

Jensen, A. R. (1969). How much can we boost IQ and scholastic achievement? *Harvard Educational Review, 39,* 1–123.

Jensen, A. R. (1973) *Educability and group differences.* London: Methuen.

Jessor, R., & Jessor, S. L. (1973). The perceived environment in behavioral science. *American Behavioral Scientist, 16,* 801–828.

Joffe, J., & Albee, G. (1981). Powerlessness and psychopathology. In J. Joffee & G. Albee (Eds.), *Prevention through political action and social change* (pp. 321–325). Hanover, NH: University Press of New England.

Jones, J. M. (1986). Racism: A cultural analysis of the problem. In J. Bovidio & S. Gaertner (Eds.), *Prejudice, discrimination, and racism.* Orlando FL: Academic Press.

Joyce, W. F., & Slocum, J. W., Jr. (1984). Collective climate: Agreement as a basis for defining climates in organizations. *Academy of Management Journal, 27,* 721–742.

Kahn, R. L., Wolfe, D. M., Quinn, R. P., Snoek, J. D., & Rosenthal, R. A. (1964). *Organizational stress: Studies in role conflict and ambiguity.* New York: Wiley.

Kalifon, Z, (1985). *Recidivism and community mental health care: A review of the literature.* Unpublished manuscript, Department of Anthropology, Northwestern University, Evanston, IL.

Kanfer, F. H., & Saslow, G. (1969). Behavioral diagnosis, In C. M. Franks (Ed.), *Behavior therapy: Appraisal and status* (pp. 417–444). New York: McGraw-Hill.

Kanner, L. (1943). Autistic disturbances of affective contact. *Nervous Child, 2*, 217–250.

Karoly, P. (Ed.). (1985). *Measurement strategies in health psychology.* New York: Wiley.

Katz, R. (1984). Empowerment and synergy: Expanding the community's healing resources. In J. Rappaport, C. Swift, & R. Hess (Eds.), *Studies in empowerment: Steps toward understanding the psychological mechanisms in preventive interventions* (pp. 201–226). New York: Haworth Press.

Katz, D., & Kahn, R. L. (1978). *The social psychology of organizations* (2nd ed.) New York: Wiley.

Kauffman, S. A. (1971). Articulation of parts explanations in biology. In R. S. Cohen & R. C. Buck (Eds.), *Boston studies in the philosophy of science: VIII* (pp. 257–272). New York: Humanities Press.

Kazdin, A. (1980). *Research design in clinical psychology.* New York: Harper & Row.

Keiffer, C. (1982). Citizen empowerment: A developmental perspective. In J. Rappaport, C. Swift, & R. Hess (Eds.) *Studies in empowerment: Steps toward understanding the psychological mechanism in preventive interventions* (pp. 9–36). New York: Haworth Press.

Keller, E. F. (1983). Gender and science. In S. Harding & M. B. Hintikka, (Eds.), *Discovering reality: Feminist perspectives on epistemology, metaphysics, methodology, and philosophy of science.* London: Reidel.

Keller, E. F. (1985) *Reflections on gender and science.* New Haven, CT.: Yale University Press.

Keller, E. F. (1987). Feminism and science. In S. Harding (Ed.), *Sex and scientific inquiry* (pp. 233–246). Chicago: University of Illinois Press.

Kelly, J. G. (1966). Ecological constraints on mental health services. *American Psychologist, 21*, 535–539.

Kelly, J. G. (1968). Toward an ecological conception of preventive interventions. In J. W. Carter, Jr. (Ed.), *Research contributions from psychology to community mental health* (pp. 75–99). New York: Behavioral Publications.

Kelly, J. G. (1970). Antidotes for arrogance: Training for a community psychology. *American Psychologist, 25*, 524–531.

Kelly, J. G. (1971). The quest for valid preventive interventions. In G. Rosenblum (Ed.), *Issues in community psychology and community mental health* (pp. 109–140). New York: Behavioral Publications.

Kelly, J. G. (1979a). *Adolescent boys in high school: A study of coping and adaptation.* Hillsdale, NJ: Erlbaum.

Kelly, J. G. (1979b). Tain't what you do, it's the way that you do it. *American Journal of Community Psychology, 7*, 239–261.

Kelly, J. G. (1984). Interpersonal and organizational resources for the continued development of community psychology. *American Journal of Community Psychology, 12*, 313–320.

Kelly, J. G. (1986a). An ecological paradigm: Defining mental health consultation as a preventative service. In J. G. Kelly & R. E. Hess (Eds.), *The ecology of prevention: Illustrating mental health consultation* (pp. 1–36). New York: Haworth Press.

Kelly, J. G. (1986b). Context and process: An ecological view of the interdependence of practice and research. *American Journal of Community Psychology, 14,* 581–589.

Kelly, J. G. (1987). Beyond prevention techniques: Creating social settings for a public's health. The Tenth Erich Lindemann Memorial Lecture, Boston, MA, April 24. (Available from J. G. Kelly, University of Illinois at Chicago, Department of Psychology).

Kelly, J. G., Altman, B. E., Kahn, R. L., Stokols, D., & Rausch, H. L. (1986). Context and process. *American Journal of Community Psychology, 14,* 573–605.

Kelly, J. G., Dassoff, N., Levin, I., Schreckengost, J., Stelzner, S. P., & Altman, B. E. (1988). *A guide to conducting prevention research in the community: First steps.* New York: Haworth Press.

Kelly, J. G., & Hess, R. E. (Eds.). (1987). *The ecology of prevention: Illustrating mental health consultation.* New York: Haworth Press.

Kelly, J. G., Ryan, A. M., & Altman, B. E. (in press). Understanding and changing social systems: An ecological view. In J. Rappaport & E. Seidman (Eds.), *Handbook of community psychology.* New York: Plenum.

Kenny, D. A. (1985). The generalized group effect model. In J. R. Nesselroade & A. von Eye (Eds.), *Individual development and social change: Exploratory analysis,* (pp. 343–357). Orlando, FL: Academic Press.

Kenny, D. A., & La Voie, L. (1985). Separating individual and group effects. *Journal of Personality and Social Psychology, 48,* 339–348.

Keys, C. B. (1988). Public interest, disciplinary interest, and the homelessness of community action. *Community Psychologist, 21,* 21–22.

Keys, C. B., & Frank, S. (1987a). Community psychology and the study of organizations: A reciprocal relationship. *American Journal of Community Psychology, 15,* 239–251.

Keys, C. B., & Frank, S. (Eds.). (1987b). Organizational perspectives in community psychology [Special issue]. *American Journal of Community Psychology, 15.*

Kieffer, C. H. (1984). Citizen empowerment: A developmental perspective. *Prevention in Human Services, 3,* 9–36.

King, Jr., M. L. (1976). The drum major instinct: A sermon to the congregation of the Ebenezer Baptist Church, Atlanta, GA. Sermon delivered February 4, 1968, and reprinted in F. Schulke (Ed.), *Martin Luther King, Jr.* (pp. 220–222). New York: Norton.

Kirkpatrick, G. (1986). *Community: A trinity of models.* Washington, DC: Georgetown University Press.

Klein, D. (1985). Afterword. In E. Susskind & D. Klein (Eds.), *Community research: Methods, paradigms and applications* (497–502). New York: Praeger.

Kornblith, H. (Ed.). (1985). *Naturalizing epistemology.* Cambridge, MA: MIT Press.

Kuhn, T. S. (1970). *The structure of scientific revolutions* (2nd ed.). Chicago: University of Chicago Press.

Lamiell, J. T. (1981). Toward an idiothetic psychology of personality. *American Psychologist, 36,* 267–289.

Lawler, E. E., Hall, D. T., & Oldham, G. R. (1974). Organizational climate: Relationship to organizational structure, process, and performance. *Organizational Behavior and Human Performance, 11,* 139–155.

Leavitt, J., & Saegert, S. (1990). *From abandonment to hope: Community households in Harlem.* New York: Columbia University Press.

Leavitt, J., & Saegert, S. (1984). Women and abandoned buildings. *Social Policy, 15*(1), 32–39.

Leplin, J. (Ed.). (1984). *Scientific realism.* Berkeley: University of California Press.

Levine, A. G. (1982). *Love Canal: Science, politics, and people.* Lexington, MA: Lexington Books.

Levine, M. (1974). Scientific method and the adversary model: Some preliminary thoughts. *American Psychologist, 29,* 661–677.

Levine, M. (1980). Investigative reporting as a research method. An analysis of Bernstein and Woodward's "All the President's Men." *American Psychologist, 35,* 626–638.

Levine, M. (1981). *The history and politics of community mental health.* New York: Oxford University Press.

Levine, M., & Levine, A. (1970). *A social history of helping services.* New York: Appleton-Century-Crofts.

Levine, M. Reppucci, N. D., & Weinstein, R. (1989). *Learning from Seymour Sarason.* Unpublished paper delivered on the occasion of Seymour B. Sarason's retirement, New Haven, CT, April 22.

Leviton, L.C., & Hughes, E. F. X. (1981). Research on the utilization of evaluations: A review and synthesis. *Evaluation Review, 5,* 525–548.

Lewin, K. (1943a). Defining the "field at a given time." *Psychological Review, 50,* 292–310.

Lewin, K. (1943b). Psychology and the process of group living. *Journal of Social Psychology, 17,* 119–129.

Lewin, K. (1951a). *Field theory in social science: Selected papers.* New York: Harper.

Lewin, K. (1951b). Frontiers in group dynamics. In D. Cartwright (Ed.), *Field theory and social science: Selected theoretical papers by Kurt Lewin.* Chicago: The University of Chicago Press. (Reprinted from *Human Relations,* 1947, *1,* 2–38)

Lewin, K. (1952). Behavior and development as a function of the total situation. In D. Cartwright (Ed.), *Field theory in social science: Selected theoretical papers by Kurt Lewin* (pp. 238–303). London: Tavistock. (Original work published in 1946)

Lewis, D., Riger, S., Wagenaar, H., Rosenbeg, H., Reed, S., & Lurigio, A. (1988). *Worlds of the mentally ill: How deinstitutionalization works in the city.* Carbondale, IL: Southern Illinois University Press.

Lidz, C. W., Mulvey, E. P., Cleveland, S., & Appelbaum, P.S. (1989). Commitment: The consistency of clinicians and the use of legal standards. *American Journal of Psychiatry, 146,* 176–181.

Lincoln, Y. S., & Guba, E. G. (1985). *Naturalistic inquiry.* Beverly Hills, CA: Sage.

Lincoln, Y. S., & Guba, E. G. (1986). But is it rigorous? Trustworthiness and authenticity in naturalistic evaluation. In *New directions for program evaluation* (Vol. 30, pp. 73–84) San Francisco: Jossey-Bass.

Lindblom, C. E. (1977). *Politics and markets: The world's political economic systems.* New York: Basic Books.

Lindblom, C. E. (1983). Comment on Manley. *American Political Science Review, 77,* 384–386.

Lindblom, C. E., & Cohen, D. K. (1979). *Usable knowledge: Social science and social problem solving.* New Haven, Connecticut: Yale University Press.

Linney, J. A. (1986). Court-ordered school desegregation: Shuffling the deck or playing a different game. In E. Seidman & J. Rappaport (Eds.), *Redefining social problems* (pp. 259–274). New York: Plenum.

Linney, J. A., & Reppucci, N. D. (1982). Research design and methods in community psychology. In P. C. Kendall & J. N. Butcher (Eds.), *Handbook of research methods in clinical psychology* (pp. 535–566). New York: Wiley.

Loo, C., Fong, K., & Iwamasa, G. (1988). Ethnicity and cultural diversity: An analysis of work published in community psychology journals, 1965–1985. *Journal of Community Psychology, 16,* 332–349.

Lopez, G., & Serrano-García, I. (1986). El poder: Posesión, capacidad o relación. *Revista de Ciencias Sociales, 25,* 121–148.

Lorion, R. P. (1983) Evaluating preventive interventions: Guidelines for the serious social change agent. In R. D. Felner, L. Jason, J. Mortisugu, & S. S. Farber (Eds.), *Preventive psychology: Theory, research and practice in community interventions.* New York: Pergamon Press.

Lorion, R. P. (1987). Methodological challenges in prevention research. In J. Steinberg & M. M. Silverman (Eds.), *Preventing mental disorders: A research perspective* (pp. 28–47). Washington, DC: U.S. Government Printing Office.

Lorion, R. P., & Allen, L. (1989). Preventive services in mental health. In D. Rochefort (Ed.), *Handbook on mental health policy in the United States* (pp. 403–434). Westport, CT: Greenwood Press.

Lorion, R. P., Bussell, D., & Goldberg, R. (in press). *Identification and assessment of youths at high-risk of substance abuse.* Washington, DC: Office of Substance Abuse Prevention, U. S. Government Printing Office.

Lorion, R. P., Cowen, E. L., & Caldwell, R. A. (1975). Normative and parametric analyses of school adjustment. *American Journal of Community Psychology, 3,* 291–301.

Lorion, R. P., Hightower, A. D., Work, W. C., & Shockley, P. (1987). The Basic Academic Skills Enhancement program: Translating prevention theory into action research. *Journal of Community Psychology, 15,* 63–77.

Lorion, R. P., Price, R. H., & Eaton, W. W. (1988). The prevention of child and adolescent disorders: From theory to research. In D. Shaffer & I. Phillips (Eds.), *Project prevention* (pp. 55–96). Washington, DC: American Academy of Child and Adolescent Psychiatry.

Lorion, R. P., Work, W. C., & Hightower, A. D. (1984). A school-based, multi-level preventive intervention: Issues in program development and evaluation. *Personnel and Guidance Journal, 62,* 479–484.

Lounsbury, J. W., Cook, M. P., Leader, D. S., & Meares, E. P. (1985). A content analysis of community psychology research. In E. C. Susskind & D. C. Klein (Eds.), *Community research: Methods, paradigms, and applications* (pp. 39–105). New York: Praeger.

Lounsbury, J., Leader, D., Meares, E., & Cook, M. (1980). An analytic review of research in community psychology. *American Journal of Community Psychology, 8,* 415–441.

Lott, B. (1985). The potential enrichment of social/personality psychology through feminist research and vice versa. *American Psychologist, 40,* 155–164.

Luepnitz, D. A. (1988a). Bateson's heritage: Bitter fruit. *The Family Systems Networker* (September/October), 49–53.

Luepnitz, D. A. (1988b). *The family interpreted: Feminist theory in clinical practice.* New York: Basic Books.

Luke, D. A. (1988). *Settings and behavior: Behavior setting theory and mutual help.* Unpublished master's thesis. University of Illinois at Urbana-Champaign.

MacIntyre, A. (1981). *After virtue.* Notre Dame. IN: University of Notre Dame Press.

Magee, B. (1973). *Karl Popper.* New York: Viking Press.

Manley, J. F. (1983). Neo-pluralism: A class analysis of Pluralism I and Pluralism II. *American Political Science Review, 77,* 368–383.

Mark, M. M., & Shortland, R. L. (1985). Stakeholder-based evaluation and value judgments. *Evaluation Review, 9,* 605–626.

Marti, S. (1980). *La identificación de necesidades como estrategia de movilización en el sector femenino del Barrio Buen Consejo.* Unpublished master's thesis. University of Puerto Rico, Rio Piedras.

Marti, S., & Serrano-García, I. (1983). Needs assessment and community development: An ideological perspective. In A. Zautra, K. Bachrach, & R. Hess (Eds.), *Strategies for needs assessment in prevention* (pp. 75–88). New York: Haworth Press.

Maruyama, M. (1983). Cross-cultural perspectives on social and community change. In E. Seidman (Ed.), *Handbook of social intervention* (pp. 33–47). Beverly Hills: CA: Sage.

Maton, K. I. (1989). Community settings as buffers of life stress? Highly supportive churches, mutual help groups, and senior centers. *American Journal of Community Psychology, 17,* 203–232.

Maton, K., & Rappaport, J. (1984). Empowerment in a religious setting: A mutlivariate investigation. *Prevention in Human Services, 3,* 37–70.

McChesney, K. Y. (1988, August). *Homelessness: A systemic problem.* Paper presented at the 96th annual convention of the American Psychological Association, Atlanta, GA.

McClure, L., Cannon, D., Belton, E., D'Ascoli, C., Sullivan, B., Allen, S., Connor, P., Stone, P., & McClure, G. (1980). Community psychology concepts and research base: Promise and product. *American Psychologist, 35,* 1000–1011.

McGrath, J. E., & Altman, I. (1966). *Small group research: A synthesis and critique of the field.* New York: Holt, Rinehart & Winston.

McGuire, W. J. (1986). The vicissitudes of attitudes and similar representational constructs in twentieth century psychology. *European Journal of Social Psychology, 16,* 89–130.

McMillan, D. W., & Chavis, D. M. (1986). Sense of community: A definition and theory. *Journal of Community Psychology, 14,* 6–23.

McVicker-Clinchy, B., & Belenky, M. F. (1987). *Women's ways of knowing: A theory and an intervention.* Speech delivered at the Day Grant Award Presentation. Smith College School of Social Work, July 23.

Meehl, P. E. (1986). What social scientists don't understand. In D. W. Fiske & R. A. Schweder (Eds.), *Metatheory in social science* (pp. 315–338). Chicago: University of Chicago Press.

Miles, M. B., & Huberman, A. M. (1984). *Qualitative data analysis: A sourcebook of new methods*. Beverly Hills, CA: Sage.

Miller, J. B. (1986). *Toward a new psychology of women* (2nd ed.) Boston: Beacon Press.

Mischler, E. G. (1979) Meaning in context: Is there any other kind? *Harvard Educational Review, 49*(1), 1–19.

Mitroff, I. (1983). Beyond experimentation: New methods for a new age. In E. Seidman (Ed.), *Handbook of social interventions* (pp. 163–177). Beverly Hills, CA.: Sage.

Moos, R. H. (1973). Conceptualizations of human environments. *American Psychologist, 28,* 652–665.

Moos, R. H. (1974). *Evaluating treatment environments: A social ecological approach.* New York: Wiley.

Moos, R. H. (1976). *The human context: Environmental determinants of behavior.* New York: Wiley.

Moos, R. H. (1984). Context and coping: Toward a unifying conceptual framework. *American Journal of Community Psychology, 12,* 5–25.

Moos, R. H. (1986). Work as a human context. In M. S. Pallak & R. O. Perloff (Eds.), *Psychology and work: Productivity, change, and employment* (pp. 9–52). Washington DC: American Psychological Association.

Moos, R. H., & Lemke, S. (1984). Supportive residential settings for older people. In I. Altman, M. P. Lawton, & J. F. Wohlwill (Eds.), *Elderly people and the environment* (pp. 159–190). New York: Plenum.

Morgan, G. (Ed). (1983). *Beyond method: Strategies for social research.* Beverly Hills, CA: Sage.

Morris, E. K. (1988). Contextualism: The world view of behavior analysis. *Journal of Experimental Child Psychology, 46,* 289–323.

Mulvey, E. P., Linney, J. A., & Rosenberg, M. (1987). Organizational control and treatment program design as dimensions of institutionalization in settings of juvenile offenders. *American Journal of Community Psychology, 15,* 321–335.

Munoz, R. F., Snowden, L. R., & Kelly, J. G. (1979). *Social and psychological research in community settings.* San Francisco: Jossey-Bass.

Murray, C. (1984). *Losing ground: American social policy, 1950–1980.* New York: Basic Books.

Murray, H. A. (1984). *Explorations in personality: A clinical and experimental study of fifty men of college age.* New York: Oxford University Press.

Murrell, S. A. (1973). *Community psychology and social systems: A conceptual framework and intervention guide.* New York: Behavioral Publications.

Naroll, R. (1983). *The moral order.* Beverly Hills, CA: Sage.

Neimann, H. T. (1987). *Predicting the quality of parent–school communication prior to kindergarten entry: Toward a systematic approach to developing effective parent–school relationships.* Unpublished doctoral dissertation, University of Tennessee, Department of Psychology.

Neruda, P. (1987). *Fully empowered.* (Bilingual ed.; Trans. Alastair Reid). New York: Farrar, Straus, & Giroux.

Nord, W. R. (1974). The failure of current applied behavioral science—A Marxian approach. *Journal of Applied Behavioral Science, 10,* 557–569.

Novaco, R., & Monahan, J. (1980). Research in community psychology: An analysis of work published in the first six years of the *American Journal of Community Psychology. American Journal of Community Psychology, 8,* 131–146.

Nunnaly, J. C. (1982). The study of human change: Measurement, research strategies, and methods of analysis. In B. B. Wolman, G. Stricker, S. J. Ellman, P. Keith-Spiegel, & D. S. Palermo (Eds.), *Handbook of developmental psychology* (pp. 133–148). Englewood Cliffs, NJ: Prentice-Hall.

Oakley, A. (1981). Interviewing women: A contradiction in terms. In H. Roberts (Ed.), *Doing feminist research.* London : Routledge & Kegan Paul.

O'Neill, P. T. H. (1989). Responsible to whom? Responsible for what? Some ethical issues in community intervention. *American Journal of Community Psychology, 17,* 323–342.

Ortiz, V. (1985). *En búsqueda de una metodología de lo cotidiano desde adentro y desde abajo.* Unpublished master's thesis. University of Puerto Rico, Rio Piedras.

Pappas, G. S., & Swain, M. (Eds.). (1978). *Essays on knowledge and justification.* London: Cornell University Press.

Parlee, M. B. (1981). Appropriate control groups in feminist research. *Psychology of Women Quarterly, 54,* 637–644.

Parsons, H. (1974). What happened at Hawthorne? *Science, 183,* 922–932.

Patton, M. Q. (1986). *Utilization-focused evaluation* (2nd ed.). Newbury Park, CA: Sage.

Patton, M. Q. (1988a). Politics and evaluation. *Evaluation Practice, 9,* 89–94.

Patton, M. Q. (1988b). The evaluator's responsibility for utilization. *Evaluation Practice, 9,* 5–24.

Pepper, S. C. (1970). *World hypotheses.* Berkeley: University of California Press.

Perry, C., & Jessor, R. (1985). The concept of health promotion and the prevention of adolescent drug abuse. *Health Education Quarterly, 12,* 169–184.

Phillips, D. D. (1976). *A systematic study of the leadership process at the corporate level of two television group owners.* Unpublished doctoral dissertation, Ohio University, Athens.

Piaget, J. (1952). *The origins of intelligence in children.* New York: Norton.

Piotrkowski, C. S. (1978). *Work and the family system: A naturalistic study of working-class and lower-middle-class families.* New York: Free Press.

Polkinghorne, D. (1983). *Methodology for the human sciences: Systems of inquiry.* Albany: State University of New York Press.

Popper, K. R. (1968). Corroboration, or how a theory stands up to tests. In K. R. Popper, *The logic of scientific discovery* (pp. 251–281). New York: Harper.

Posavac, E. J., & Carey, R. G. (1989). *Program evaluation: Methods and case studies* (3rd ed.). Englewood Cliffs, NJ: Prentice Hall.

Powell-Hopson, D., & Hopson, D. (1989). *Reflections of racism: Implications of doll color preferences among Black preschool children and White preschool children.* Unpublished manuscript.

Price, R. H. (1988, August). *Bearing witness.* Distinguished Contribution Award Address, to the Division of Community Psychology, delivered at the 96th annual convention of the American Psychological Association, Atlanta, GA.

Price, R. H., Cowen, E. L., Lorion, R. P., & Ramos-McKay, J. (Eds.). (1988). *14 ounces of prevention: A casebook for practitioners.* Washington, DC: American Psychological Association.

Proshansky, H. M., Ittelson, W. H., & Rivlin, L. G. (1970). The influence of the physical environment on behavior: Some basic assumptions. In H. M. Proshansky, W. H. Ittelson, & L. G. Rivlin (Eds.), *Environmental psychology: Man and his physical setting* (pp. 27–37). New York: Holt, Rinehart & Winston.

Quattrochi-Tubin, S., & Jason, L. A. (1980). Enhancing social interactions and activity among the elderly through stimulus control. *Journal of Applied Behavior Analysis, 13,* 159–163.

Quine W. V., & Ullian, J. S. (1970). *The web of belief* (2nd ed). New York: Random House.

Ramirez, M. (1983). *Psychology of the Americas: Multicultural perspectives in personality and mental health.* New York: Pergamon Press.

Rapkin, B. D. (1985). *Multidimensional scaling of outcome domains in an intervention for nursing home residents.* Unpublished master's thesis, University of Illinois at Urbana-Champaign.

Rappaport, J. (1977). *Community psychology: Values, research and action.* New York: Holt, Rinehart & Winston.

Rappaport, J. (1981). In praise of paradox: A social policy of empowerment over prevention. *American Journal of Community Psychology, 9,* 1–25.

Rappaport, J. (1984). Seeking justice in the real world: A further explication of value contexts. *Journal of Community Psychology, 12,* 208–216.

Rappaport, J. (1985). The power of empowerment language. *Social Policy, 16,* 15–21.

Rappaport, J. (1987). Terms of empowerment/exemplars of prevention: Toward a theory of community psychology. *American Journal of Community Psychology, 15,* 121–148.

Rappaport, J., Davidson, W. S., Wilson, M., & Mitchell, A. (1975). Alternatives to blaming the victim or the environment: Our places to stand have not moved the earth. *American Psychologist, 30,* 525–528.

Rappaport, J., Seidman, E., & Davidson, W. S. (1979). Demonstration research and manifest versus true adoption: The natural history of a research project to divert adolescents from the legal system. In R. F. Munoz, L. R. Snowden, & J. G. Kelly (Eds.), *Social and psychological research in community settings* (pp. 101–144). San Francisco: Jossey-Bass.

Rappaport, J., Seidman, E., Toro, P., McFadden, L. S., Reischl, T. M., Roberts, L. J., Salem, D. A., Stein, C. H., & Zimmerman, M. A. (1985). Collaborative research with a mutual help organization. *Social Policy, 15,* 12–24.

Reinharz, S. (1979). *On becoming a social scientist: From survey research and participant observation to experiential analysis.* San Francisco: Jossey-Bass.

Reinharz, S. (1984). Women as competent community builders: The other side of the coin. In A. U. Rickel, M. Gerrard, & I. Iscoe (Eds.), *Social and psychological problems of women.* New York: Hemisphere.

Reinharz, S. (1988, October). *The concept of voice.* Paper presented at conference "Human Diversity: Perspectives on People in Context," held at the University of Maryland, College Park.

Repetti, R. L. (1987). Individual and common components of the social environment at work and psychological well-being. *Journal of Personality and Social Psychology, 52,* 710–720.

Rescher, N. (1969). *Introduction to value theory.* Englewood Cliffs, NJ: Prentice-Hall.

Riegel, K. F. (1976). The dialectics of human development. *American Psychologist, 31,* 689–700.

Riger, S., & Keys, C. (1987, May). *Feminist organizations as organized anarchies: A portrait of consensus decision making in action.* Paper presented at the First Biennial Community Psychology conference, held in Charleston, SC.

Roberts, K. H., Hulin, C. L., & Rousseau, D. M. (1978). *Developing an interdisciplinary science of organizations,* San Francisco: Jossey-Bass.

Robinson, W. S. (1950). Ecological correlations and the behavior of individuals. *American Sociological Review, 15,* 351–357.

Rodriguez, R. (1982). *Hunger of memory: The education of Richard Rodriguez.* New York: Bantam.

Roethlisberger, F. J. (1977). *The elusive phenomena: An autobiographical account of my work in the field of organized behavior at the Harvard Business School.* Cambridge, MA: Harvard University, Division of Research, Graduate School of Business Administration (distributed by Harvard University Press).

Rosario, W. (1984). *El desarrollo de comunidad y la promoción popular como vehículos liberadores ante la marginalización.* Unpublished master's thesis. University of Puerto Rico, Rio Piedras.

Rose, H. (1987). Hand, brain, and heart: A feminist epistemology for the natural sciences. In S. Harding (Ed.), *Sex and scientific inquiry* (pp. 265–282). Chicago: University of Illinois Press.

Rosnow, R. L., & Georgoudi, M. (1986). The spirit of contextualism. In R. L. Rosnow & M. Georgoudi (Eds.), *Contextualism and understanding in behavioral science: Implications for research and theory* (pp. 3–22). New York: Praeger.

Rothman, J., & Tropman, J. E. (1987). Models of community organization and macro practice perspectives: Their mixing and phasing. In F. M. Cox, J. L. Erlich, J. Rothman, & J. E. Tropman (Eds.), *Strategies of community organization: Macropractice* (4th Ed., pp. 3–26). Itasca, IL: Peacock.

Rotter, J. B. (1954). *Social learning and clinical psychology.* Englewood Cliffs, NJ: Prentice-Hall.

Rousseau, D. M. (1985). Issues of level in organizational research: Multi-level and cross-level perspectives. In L. L. Cummings & B. M. Staw (Eds.), *Research in organizational behavior* (Vol. 7, pp. 1–37). Greenwich, CT: JAI Press.

Ruback, R. B., & Innes, C. A. (1988). The relevance and irrelevance of psychological research: The example of prison crowding. *American Psychologist, 43,* 683–693.

Runyan, W. M. (1984). *Life histories and psychobiography: Explorations in theory and method.* New York: Oxford University Press.

Russell, B. (1945). *The history of western philosophy.* New York: Simon & Schuster.

Ryan, W. (1971). *Blaming the victim.* New York: Vintage Books.

Salem, D. A. (1988). *The measurement of community adjustment: An ecological perspective.* Unpublished doctoral dissertation, University of Illinois at Urbana–Champaign.

Sameroff, A. J., & Chandler, M. J. (1975). Reproductive risk and the continuum of caretaking casualty. In F. D. Horowitz, M. Hetherington, S. Scarr-Salapatek, & G. Siegel (Eds.), *Review of child development research* (Vol. 4). Chicago: University of Chicago Press.

Sameroff, A. J., & Fiese, B. (1988) Conceptual issues in prevention. In D. Shaffer & I. Phillips (Eds.), *Project prevention*. Washington, DC: American Academy of Child and Adolescent Psychiatry.

Sandler, I. N., & Keller, P. A. (1984). Trends observed in community psychology training descriptions. *American Journal of Community Psychology, 12,* 157–164.

Santiago, L., & Perfecto, G. (1983). *Hacia el encuentro de la psicología social comunitaria y el cristianismo en un esfuerzo investigativo con énfasis en la partricipación comunitaria.* Unpublished master's thesis. University of Puerto Rico, Rio Piedras.

Santostefano, S. (1978). *A biodevelopmental approach to clinical child psychology.* New York: Wiley.

Sarason, S. B. (1972). *The creation of settings and the future societies.* San Francisco, CA: Jossey-Bass.

Sarason, S. B. (1974). *The psychological sense of community: Prospects for the community psychology.* San Francisco: Jossey-Bass.

Sarason, S. B. (1976). Psychology to the Finland Station in the heavenly city of the eighteenth century philosophers. *American Psychologist, 30,* 1072–1080.

Sarason, S. B. (1978). The nature of problem solving in social action. *American Psychologist, 33,* 370–380.

Sarason, S. B. (1981). *Psychology misdirected.* New York: Free Press.

Sarason, S. B. (1982a). *The culture of the school and the problem of change.* (2nd ed.). Boston: Allyn & Bacon.

Sarason, S. B. (1982b). *Psychology and social action: Selected papers.* New York: Praeger.

Sarason, S. B. (1988). *The making of an American psychologist. An autobiography.* San Francisco: Jossey-Bass.

Sarason, S. B., Carroll, C., Maton, K., Cohen, S., & Lorentz, E. (1977). *Human services and resource networks.* San Francisco: Jossey-Bass.

Sarason, S. B., & Doris, J. (1979). *Education handicap, public policy and social history.* New York: Free Press.

Sarason, I. G., Johnson, J. H., & Siegel, J. M. (1978). Assessing the impact of life changes: Development of the Life Experiences Survey. *Journal of Consulting and Clinical Psychology, 46,* 932–946.

Sarbin, T. R. (1970). A role theory perspective for community psychology: The structure of social identity. In D. Adelson & B. L. Kalis (Eds.), *Community psychology and mental health: Perspectives and challenges* (pp. 89–113). Scranton, PA: Chandler.

Scheff, T. J. (1966). *Being mentally ill: A sociological theory.* Chicago: Aldine.

Scheirer, M. A. (1987). Program theory and implementation theory: Implications for evaluators. In L. Bickman (Ed.), *Using program theory in evaluation.* San Francisco: Jossey-Bass.

Schneider, B., & Reichers, A. E. (1983). On the etiology of climates. *Personnel Psychology, 36,* 19–39.

Schoggen, P. (1989). *Behavior settings: A revision and extension of Roger C. Barker's ecological psychology.* Stanford, CA: Stanford University Press.

Schrag, C. O. (1988). Liberal learning in the postmodern world. *Key Reporter, 54,* 1-4.

Schriner, K. F., & Fawcett, S. B. (1988). Development and validation of a community concerns reports method. *Journal of Community Psychology, 16,* 306-316.

Scriven, M. (1980). *The logic of evaluation.* Inverness, CA: Edgepress.

Seekins, T., & Fawcett, S. B. (1984). Planned diffusion of social technologies for community groups. In S. C. Paine, G. T. Bellamy, & B. Wilcox (Eds.), *Human services that work: From innovation to standard practice* (pp. 247-260). Baltimore, MD: Paul H. Brookes.

Seekins, T., & Fawcett, S. B. (1987). Effects of a poverty-clients agenda on resource allocations by community decision makers. *American Journal of Community Psychology, 15,* 305-320.

Seekins, T., Maynard-Moody, S., & Fawcett, S. B. (1987). Understanding the policy process: Preventing and coping with community problems. In L. A. Jason, R. E. Hess, R. D. Felner, & J. N. Moritsugu (Eds.), *Prevention: Toward a multidisciplinary approach* (pp. 65-89). New York: Haworth Press.

Seidman, E. (1978). Justice, values and social science: Unexamined premises. In R. J. Simon (Ed.), *Research in law and sociology* (pp. 175-200). Greenwich, CT: JAI Press.

Seidman, E. (1983). Unexamined premises of social problem solving. In E. Seidman (Ed.), *Handbook of social intervention* (pp. 48-67). Beverly Hills: Sage.

Seidman, E. (1987). Toward a framework for primary prevention research. In J. A. Steinberg & M. M. Silverman (Eds.), *Preventing mental disorders: A research perspective* (pp. 2-19). Washington, DC: U.S. Government Printing Office.

Seidman, E. (1988). Back to the future, community psychology: Unfolding a theory of social intervention. *American Journal of Community Psychology, 16,* 3-24.

Seidman, E., & Rapkin, B. (1983). Economics and psychosocial dysfunction: Toward a conceptual framework and prevention strategies. In R. D. Felner, L. A. Jason, J. N. Moritsugu, & S. S. Farber (Eds.), *Preventive psychology: Theory, research, and practice* (pp. 175-198). New York: Pergamon.

Seidman, E., & Rappaport, J. (1986). *Redefining social problems.* New York: Plenum.

Sennet, R., & Cobb, J. (1973). *The hidden injuries of class.* New York: Vintage.

Serrano-García, I. (1984). The illusion of empowerment: Community development within a colonial context. In J. Rappaport, C. Swift, & R. Hess (Eds.), *Studies in empowerment: Steps toward understanding and action* (pp. 173-200). New York: Haworth Press.

Serrano-García, I. (in press). Intervención en la investigación: Su desarrollo. In I. Serrano-García (Ed.), *Contribuciones puertoriqueñas a la psicologia social-comunitaria.* Rio Piedras, PR: Editorial Universitaria.

Serrano-García, I., Lopez, M. M., & Rivera-Medina, E. (1987). Toward a social-community psychology. *Journal of Community Psychology, 15*(4), 431-446.

Serrano-García, I., Suarez, A., Alvarez, S., & Rosario, W. (1980, July). *El Proyecto Buen Consejo: Un escenario de adiestramiento y cambio social.* Paper presented at the 1st Latin American Congress of Psychology in the Community, Havana, Cuba.

Shadish, W. R. (1984). Policy research: Lessons from the implementation of deinstitution-alization. *American Psychology, 39,* 725–738.

Shadish, W. R. (1986a). Planned critical multiplism: Some elaborations. *Behavioral Assessment, 8,* 75–103.

Shadish, W. R. (1986b). Sources of evaluation practice: Needs, purposes, questions, and technology. In L. Bickman & D. L. Weatherford (Eds.), *Evaluating early intervention programs for severely handicapped children and their families* (pp. 149–183). Austin, TX: Pro-Ed.

Shadish, W. R. (1987). Program micro- and macrotheories: A guide for social change. In L. Bickman (Ed.), *Using program theory in evaluation* (pp. 93–109). San Francisco: Jossey-Bass.

Shadish, W. R. (1989). Critical multiplism: A research strategy and its attendant tactics. In L. Sechrest, H. Freeman, & A. Mulley (Eds.), *Health services research methodology: A focus on AIDS* (pp. 5–28). (OHHS Pub. No. PHS-89-3439). Rockville, MD: National Center for Health Services Research and Health Care Technology Assessment, Public Health Service, U.S. Department of Health and Human Services.

Shadish, W. R., Cook, T. D., & Houts, A. C. (1986). Quasiexperimentation in a critical multiplist mode. *New Directions for Program Evaluation, 31,* 29–46.

Shadish, W. R., & Epstein, R. (1987). Patterns of program evaluation practice among members of the Evaluation Research Society and Evaluation Network. *Evaluation Review, 11,* 555–590.

Shapiro, B. J. (1983). *Probability and certainty in seventeenth-century England: A study of the relationships between natural science, religion, history, law, and literature.* Princeton, NJ: Princeton University Press.

Sherif, C. (1987). Bias in psychology. In S. Harding (Ed.), *Feminism and methodology: Social science issues* (pp. 37–56). Bloomington: Indiana University Press.

Sherif, M. (1936). *The psychology of social norms.* New York: Harper.

Shinn, M. (1978). Father absence and children's cognitive development. *Psychological Bulletin, 85,* 295–324.

Shinn, M., Morich, H., Robinson, P. E., & Neuner, R. A. (1986). *Coping with job stress: Individual, group, and organizational strategies.* Unpublished manuscript, New York University.

Shinn, M., & Perkins, D. (in press). Contributions from organizational psychology. In J. Rappaport & E. Seidman (Eds.), *The handbook of community psychology.*

Shinn, M., Rosario, M., Morch, H., & Chestnut, D. E. (1984). Coping with job stress and burnout in the human services. *Journal of Personality and Social Psychology, 46,* 864–876.

Shweder, R. A. (1986). Divergent rationalities. In D. W. Fiske & R. A. Shweder (Eds.), *Metatheory in social science: Pluralisms and subjectives* (pp. 163–196). Chicago: University of Chicago Press.

Skinner, B. F. (1953). *Science and human behavior.* New York: Free Press.

Slavin, R. E. (1983). *Cooperative learning.* New York: Longman.

Solano, R. (1979). *Detección de necesidades en la comunidad rural La Plata en Albonito.* Unpublished master's thesis, University of Puerto Rico, Rio Piedras.

Special feature: Participatory Research (1975). *Convergence, 8,* 24–87.

Sroufe, L. A., & Rutter, M. (1984) The domain of developmental psychopathology. *Child Development, 55,* 17–29.

Stake, R. E. (1986). *Quieting reform*. Urbana: University of Illinois Press.

Staw, B. M., Sandelands, L. E., & Dutton, J. E. (1981). Threat rigidity effects in organizational behavior: A multilevel analysis. *Administrative Science Quarterly, 26*, 501–524.

Stern, G. G. (1970). *People in context: Measuring person–environment congruence in education and industry*. New York: Wiley.

Suárez, A. (1985). *La dinámica de grupos en reuniónes de líderes de una comunidad puertorriqueña*. Unpublished master's thesis, University of Puerto Rico, Rio Piedras.

Suppe, F. (1974). *The structure of scientific theories* (2nd ed). Chicago: University of Illinois Press.

Susskind, E. (1985). A multiparadigmatic approach to community research: Paradigm choice, experiential validity and commitment. In E. C. Susskind & D. C. Klein (Eds.), *Community research: Methods, paradigms, and applications* (pp. 5–38). New York: Praeger.

Susskind, E. C., & Klein, D. C. (Eds.). (1985). *Community research: Methods, paradigms, and applications*. New York: Praeger.

Swift, C. (1986). Community intervention in sexual child abuse. In S. Auerbach & A. Stolberg (Eds.), *Crisis intervention with children and families* (pp. 149–172). Washington, DC: Hemisphere.

Swift, C., & Levin, G. (1987). Empowerment: An emerging mental health technology. *Journal of Primary Prevention, 7*(3), 242–263.

Tannenbaum, A. S. (1974). *Hierarchy in organizations*. San Francisco: Jossey-Bass.

Taylor, S. T., & Bogdan, R. (1984). *Introduction to qualitative research methods: The search for meanings* (2nd ed.). New York: Wiley.

Tolan, P. H. (1987). Delinquent behaviors and male adolescent development: A preliminary study. *Journal of Youth and Adolescence, 17*, 413–427.

Trickett, E. J. (1984). Toward a distinctive community psychology: An ecological metaphor for the conduct of community research and the nature of training. *American Journal of Community Psychology, 12*, 261–279.

Trickett, E. J., & Birman, D. (1987). Taking ecology seriously: A community development approach to individually based preventive interventions in schools. In L. Bond & B. Compas (Eds.), *Primary prevention and promotion in the schools* (pp. 361–390). Beverly Hills, CA: Sage.

Trickett, E. J., Kelly, J. G., & Todd, D. M. (1972). The social environment of the high school: Guidelines for individual change and organizational development. In S. G. Golann & Eisdorfer (Eds.), *Handbook of community mental health* (pp. 331–406). New York: Appleton-Century-Crofts.

Trickett, E. J., Kelly, J. G., & Vincent, T. (1985). The spirit of ecological inquiry in community research. In E. Susskind & D. Klein (Eds.), *Community research: Methods, paradigms, and applications* (pp. 5–38). New York: Praeger.

Trickett, E. J., & Mitchell, R. E. (in press). An ecological metaphor for research and intervention in community psychology. In M. S. Gibbs, J. R. Lachenmeyer, & J. Sigal (Eds.), *Community psychology: Theoretical and empirical approaches* (2nd ed.). New York: Wiley.

Tukey, J. W. (1977). *Exploratory data analysis*. Reading, MA: Addison-Wesley.

U.S. Bureau of Census (1986). *Census data*. Washington, DC: U.S. Government Printing Office.

van Bertanlanffy, L. (1968). General systems theory: Foundation, developments, applications. New York: Braziller.

Van Mannen, J. (Ed.). (1983). Qualitative methodology. Beverly Hills, CA: Sage.

Van Mannen, J., Dabbs, J. M., Jr., & Faulkner, R. R. (1982). Varieties of qualitative
research. Beverly Hills, CA: Sage.

Videka, L. (1979). Psychosocial adaptation in a medical self-help group. In M. A.
Lieberman, L. Borman, & Associates (Eds.), Self-help groups for coping with crisis
(pp. 362–386). San Francisco: Jossey-Bass.

Vincent, T. A., & Trickett, E. J. (1983). Preventive interventions and the human context:
Ecological approaches to environmental assessment and change. In R. D. Felner,
L. A. Jason, J. N. Moritsugu, & S. S. Farber (Eds.), Preventive psychology: Theory,
research, and practice (pp. 67–86). New York: Pergamon Press.

Von Eckartsberg, R. (1985). Existential–phenomenological knowledge building. In E.
Susskind & D. Klein (Eds.), Community research: Methods, paradigms, and applications (pp. 334–359). New York: Praeger.

Wagner, J. (1987). The search for signs of intelligent life in the universe. New York:
Harper & Row.

Wallston, B. S. (1981). What are the questions in the psychology of women? A feminist
approach to research. Psychology of Women Quarterly, 5(4), 597–617.

Walsh, M. R. (Ed.). (1987). The psychology of women: Ongoing debates. New Haven,
CT: Yale University Press.

Walsh, R. T. (1987a). A social historical note on the formal emergence of community
psychology. American Journal of Community Psychology, 15, 523–529.

Walsh, R. T. (1987b). The evolution of the research relationship in community psychology.
American Journal of Community Psychology, 15, 773–788.

Wandersman, A., Florin, P., Friedmann, R., & Meier, R. (1987). Who participates, who
does not, and why? An analysis of voluntary neighborhood organizations in the United
States and Israel. Sociological Forum, 2, 534–555.

Warwick, D. P., & Kelman, H. C. (1976). Ethical issues in social intervention. In W. G.
Bennis, K. D. Benne, R. Chin, & K. E. Corey (Eds.), The planning of change (3rd
ed., pp. 470–496). New York: Holt, Rinehart & Winston.

Warwick, D., & Lininger, C. (1975). The sample survey: Theory and practice. New York:
McGraw-Hill.

Watzlawick, P., Weakland, J. H., & Fisch, R. (1974). Change: Principles of problem
formation and problem resolution. New York: Norton.

Webb, E. J., Campbell, D. T., Schwartz, R. D., Sechrest, L., & Grove, J. B. (1981).
Nonreactive measures in the social sciences (2nd ed.). Boston: Houghton Mifflin.

Wechsler, H., & Pugh, T. F. (1967). Fit of individual and community characteristics and
rates of psychiatric hospitalization. American Journal of Sociology, 73, 331–338.

Weick, K. E. (1984). Small wins: Redefining the scale of social problems. American
Psychologist, 39, 40–49.

Weiss, C. H. (1978). Improving the linkage between social research and public policy. In
L. E. Lynn (Ed.), Knowledge and policy: The uncertain connection (pp. 23–81).
Washington, DC: National Academy of Sciences.

Weiss, C. H. (1988). Evaluation for decisions: Is anybody there? Does anybody care?
Evaluation Practice, 9, 5–20.

Weiss, C. H., & Bucuvalas, M. J. (1980). *Social science research and decision making.* New York: Columbia University Press.

Wellman, B., & Berkowitz, S. D. (1988). Introduction: Studying social structures. In B. Wellman & S. D. Berkowitz (Eds.), *Social structures: A network approach* (pp. 1–14). Cambridge, England: Cambridge University Press.

Westkott, M. (1979). Feminist criticism of the social sciences. *Harvard Educational Review, 49*(4), 422–430.

Wholey, S. S. (1983). Evaluation and effective public management. Boston: Little, Brown.

Whyte, W. F. (1943). *Street corner society.* Chicago: University of Chicago Press.

Whyte, W. F. (1948). *Human relations in the restaurant industry.* New York: McGraw-Hill.

Wicker, A. W. (1972). Processes which mediate behavior–environment congruence. *Behavioral Science, 17,* 265–277.

Wicker, A. W. (1984). *An introduction to ecological psychology.* New York: Cambridge University Press. (Original work published 1979)

Wicker, A. W. (1985). Getting out of our conceptual ruts: Strategies for expanding our conceptual frameworks. *American Psychologist, 40,* 1094–1103.

Wicker, A. W. (1986, August). *Substantive theorizing: Clothing for a naked emperor?* Paper presented at the 94th annual convention of the American Psychological Association, Washington, DC

Wicker, A. W. (1987). Behavior settings reconsidered: Temporal stages, resources, internal dynamics, context. In D. Stokols & I. Altman (Eds.), *Handbook of environmental psychology* (pp. 613–653). New York: Wiley.

Wicker, A. W., McGrath, J. E., & Armstrong, G. E. (1972). Organization size and behavior setting capacity as determinants of member participation. *Behavioral Science, 17,* 499–513.

Wimsatt, W. C. (1974). Complexity and organization. In K. F. Schaffner & R. S. Cohen (Eds.), *Proceedings of the meetings of the Philosophy of Science Association, 1972.* Dordrecht, Netherlands: Reidel.

Wimsatt, W. C. (1981). Robustness, reliability, and over-determination. In M. Brewer & B. Collins (Eds.), *Scientific inquiry and the social sciences* (pp. 124–163). San Francisco: Jossey-Bass.

Winnett, R. A., Lecklitter, I. N., Chinn, D. E., Stahl, B., & Love S. (1985). Effects of television modeling on residential energy conservation. *Journal of Applied Behavior Analysis, 18,* 33–44.

Wofford, J. C., & Srinivasan, T. N. (1983). Experimental tests of the leader-environment-follower interaction theory of leadership. *Organizational Behavior and Human Performance, 32,* 35–54.

Wolf, M. M. (1978). Social validity: The case for subjective measurement or how applied behavior analysis is finding its heart. *Journal of Applied Behavior Analysis, 11,* 203–214.

Wolff, T. (1987). Community psychology and empowerment: An activist insight. *American Journal of Community Psychology, 15,* 151–166.

Wood, J. V., Taylor, S. E., & Lichtman, R. R. (1985). Social comparison in adjustment to breast cancer. *Journal of Personality and Social Psychology, 49,* 1169–1183.

Yin, R. K. (1985). *Case study research.* Beverly Hills, CA: Sage.

Zane, N. L., & Sue, S. (1986). Reappraisal of ethnic minority issues: Research alternatives. In E. Seidman & J. Rappaport (Eds.), *Redefining social problems* (pp. 289–
304). New York: Plenum.

Zautra, A., Bachrach, K., & Hess, R. (Eds.) (1983). *Strategies for needs assessment in
prevention.* New York: Haworth Press.

Zeiler, M. D. (1978). Principles of behavior control. In T. A. Brigham & A. C. Catania
(Eds.), *Handbook of applied behavior analysis* (pp. 17–60). New York: Irvington.

INDEX